Praise for
You're Not Crazy and You're Not Alone

"I've read most of the Thyroid / Hashimoto's books out there and have gained a well-rounded education on all the best ways to manage it, but this book is different... *You're Not Crazy and You're Not Alone* delves into the emotions behind those with Hashimoto's. This hit home to me as someone who's always strongly felt that my Hashimoto's was at least partially triggered by emotional stress. Stacey has written a poignant, emotionally-stirring account of her journey with Hashimoto's, which also serves to put us in touch with our own emotions and how they play a role in our health and wellbeing. Our members of the Hashimoto's 411 group have always given Stacey's writings positive feedback and they've always begged for more in the form of a book - she has definitely delivered!"

Alice McDonnell
Founder of Hashimotos411 and Hashimoto's patient

"*You're Not Crazy and You're Not Alone* is a gateway to the deeper understanding of health and well-being mentally, spiritually and physically, whilst living with Hashimoto's disease. A *must read* for everyone who is either just starting their autoimmune journey, or is well on their way to wellness. This amazing collection of wisdom will benefit everyone who reads it. Stacey writes from almost two decades of experience, and writes it in a way that is easy to take in (yes, even if you still have brain fog!). It will make you laugh at times, but may also make you cry with the understanding and depth she shares with a huge amount grace and love. The knowledge shared in this book can save you having to learn many lessons the hard way, and let's face it, living with Hashimoto's can be hard enough! I only wish this book was available at the beginning of my journey!"

Danielle Pearsall
Thyroid Advocate (Australia)

"Well-written from a well-informed and brilliant consumer, this enlightening book not only depicts a woman with an autoimmune disease desperately seeking help, but also details the many contributing life factors, as well as experiences with clinicians who have, over the years, belittled her symptoms and ignored her cries for help. However, you won't find that Mrs. Robbins dwells on the negative; instead, she focuses on the positive and the greatness of this thing called life. This is a wonderful, candid and easy read that will evoke a multitude of emotions from the reader: laughter, gratitude, appreciation, empowerment, more laughter, frustration, compassion, the discovery of truth, empathy, and of course, more laughter. As a medical provider with Hashimoto's, I found myself nodding in agreement, shaking my head acknowledging the painful reality of true lack of knowledge within my field, as well as my eyebrows raising when met with new information and issues I'd never considered. This is a true eye-opener for anyone with Hashimoto's..."

Paige Adams, FNP, B-C
www.proactivemed.org

"Stacey is a true gem! She has been given the ability to deeply express how life traumas and victories shape our world-view and ultimately our lives. This is comforting news because many who experience life traumas lack the courage, language or voice to process their pain into something wonderful and liberating. Her candor and her compassion will set you at ease in the same way that a trusted friend can be relied upon to protect your shame and walk beside you to a place of peace and understanding."

Ralph Umbriaco D.C.

"A brutally honest look at one woman's inspiring journey to healing from Hashimoto's - not only physically, but soul deep. I saw myself in every sorrow and every struggle, and that gave me hope that I will see myself in the joy and healing, too. It was like having Stacey right there with me holding my hand through some of the darkest times in my life and I knew I wasn't crazy and I really wasn't alone."

Sara Lunsford, author of
***Sweet Hell on Fire* and Hashimoto's patient**

"Stacey has written a much needed book for those suffering with Hashimoto's and the doctors that care for them. She sheds light on the psychology of being sick and how to gently love ourselves back to better. All doctors should strive to better understand their patients' experience. This will help them approach their patients from a place of compassion, non-judgment and work with them from 'where they are at.'"

Koren Barrett N.D.
www.npihealth.com

"What you hold in your hands is a very personal journey through life with an autoimmune label. The reader will find much of their own story in Stacey's as we find there is universal commonalities in all Hashimoto's or autoimmune people. Every chapter entertains, educates and elucidates the path that we all go or will go through as we heal from autoimmune or any chronic illness. The stories and strategies will resonate with the reader on many levels. *You're Not Crazy and You're Not Alone* is the "Hitchhiker's Guide to the Hashimoto's Universe" – every bit as funny and sad, poignant and purposeful so, at the end of the book you should be left with hope and direction. What a wonderful resource we now have."

Brett Jacques N.D.
www.newportlongevitycenter.com

"Author, Stacey Robbins, has done something wonderful in her new book, *You're Not Crazy and You're Not Alone.* She has helped humanize and bring to light many of the internal struggles that are so much a part of chronic diseases like Hashimoto's. The emotional, psychological and self-esteem issues of dealing with this difficult health disorder are illustrated with humor, compassion and hope. This is a must read for anyone who really wants to heal."

Marc Ryan, L.Ac.
Founder of www.hashimotoshealing.com

"A touching affirmation of hope, faith and healing."

Tara West
Amazon bestselling author & Hashimoto's patient

"How can one person deal with so much tragedy, disappointment, and the worst of all abuses and come out as an inspiration with a beguiling sense of humor? In Stacey Robbins' latest
book *You're Not Crazy and You're Not Alone* she shares her story
of personal triumphs that would have crushed most people. But
Stacey has a way of turning a negative into a positive. Whether or not you're familiar with Hashimoto's disease, and hopeful-
ly you've never heard of it, you'll benefit from reading Stacey's
journey that can bring hope and light to anyone going through
hardships and dismal events. We need more people like Stacey
who can provide insight and inspiration when life's issues seem
insurmountable."

Greer Wylder
Founder and Editor, Greer's OC

"Stacey writes as if speaking to a longtime friend in a voice so
refreshingly straightforward and truthful, you'll find yourself completely enthralled in her story. Reading this book is akin to having
an enlightened conversation with a witty and humorous sage. But
best of all, the take away from her life/health experiences, shared
with no holds barred, are the sensible, easy-to-implement anti-
dotes to symptoms that have stymied so many of us who have
been given a diagnosis of Hashimoto's."

Irene Dunlap, Co-author
***Chicken Soup for the Soul* book series**

"As a person who has lived with very close family members with
an autoimmune disease, I was completely amazed at how I could
see each of them in many different ways within this book. As a
woman, I was completely amazed at how I could see myself in
many different ways within this book...and I do not have Hashimoto
Disease. Stacey's insights and wisdom come to life through the
Love she so beautifully pens for the healing of others. This book
is a call out of the shadows to the parts of the heart where needed....for anyone who reads it!"

Carol A. Meadors, M. A.,
Licensed Professional Counselor at Life Focus, Inc.

Also by Stacey Robbins:

Bloom Beautiful
Inspiration for the Soul

Original quotes by Stacey Robbins
Designs by Susannah Parrish

www.bloombeautiful.com

You're Not Crazy
and
You're Not Alone

Losing the Victim, Finding Your Sense of Humor, and Learning to Love Yourself through Hashimoto's

By Stacey Robbins

You're Not Crazy and You're Not Alone
Losing the Victim, Finding Your Sense of Humor, and Learning to Love Yourself through Hashimoto's

First printing, 2013

Library of Congress Control Number: 2013919807
ISBN 978-0-615-91276-9

Stacey Robbins
427 East 17th Street Box 123
Costa Mesa, CA 92627
www.staceyrobbins.com

Disclaimer: This book is intended to be an inspiring companion to your inner healing journey, offering encouragement and empowerment to the reader. This book is not intended as a substitute for psychological treatment or the medical advice of physicians and other health professionals. The reader should regularly consult a physician in matters relating to his/her health and particularly with respect to any symptoms that may require diagnosis or medical attention.

Cover and Interior Layout and Design:
David Trotter (www.8trackstudios.com)

Back Cover Photo:
Rock Robbins and Nigel Skeet (www.nigelskeet.com)

Dedication

This book is dedicated with love and compassion:

To all the women who feel like they got blindsided with an autoimmune dis-ease and feel like they can't go one more day.

I believe you've drawn this book to you because you're ready to take your life to the next healing level. It is here to remind you that healing is possible, that you're not always going to feel this way, and that Wisdom is a breath way.

I'm here to remind you that you're not crazy.

and

To all the people: Family, friends, doctors, healers, lovers and angelic strangers who care for someone with these mostly invisible, but painful issues that come along with Hashimoto's.

Thank you for being there in a way that no one else is. Your love holds a special place in our heart and our healing. We cherish you, even though we're cranky with you. Thank you for not taking us personally and yet being so personally invested. Thank you for holding on to us when we stopped holding onto hope. Thank you for giving us love while we are still learning how to receive it.

You remind us that we're not alone.

This book is sent with love, healing and gratitude to you all.

Contents

Foreword

When I was first diagnosed with Hashimoto's in 2009, I set out on a journey to discover the root cause of my condition by figuring out the lifestyle factors and triggers that led me and other genetically susceptible individuals to develop this condition. As many of you may know, not everyone with the same genes gets Hashimoto's. There has to be a triggering event or series of events that results in gene expression.

I used my background as a pharmacist to comb through the emerging scientific literature available on autoimmunity and tested various interventions on myself to find my own root cause.

I have always been keen on recognizing patterns, and speaking with other Hashimoto's patients allowed me to connect the dots to my own condition. Many of us with Hashimoto's have had acid reflux, a history of irritable bowel syndrome, and other gut problems. Some of us also presented with anemia, anxiety and low blood pressure. I used these commonalities to figure out a way to break the vicious cycle of my Hashimoto's, though identifying and correcting food sensitivities, gut infections and adrenal problems.

The more I dug into the world of healing and into speaking with other patients, the more I realized the impact of one particular trigger...stress.

Literature reviews as well as personal conversations with many of those with Hashimoto's revealed that stress is often a precursor for autoimmunity. Many people have been able to pinpoint the beginning of their symptoms to a particularly difficult life event.

But stress isn't always external or a one time deal. Chronic stress can also play a role in autoimmune disease, and this type of stress often comes from within, in how we interpret and perceive the world. In speaking with other thyroid patients, it came to my attention that many of us also share some personality traits that include having a Type A personality, fear of failure, perfectionism, negative self-talk and generally being very tough on ourselves.

Learning to accept myself and letting go of wanting to be perfect was a major part of my healing journey. My book, "Hashimoto's Thyroiditis: Lifestyle Interventions for Finding and Treating the Root Cause" is a testament of my self-acceptance. The old me would have never been able to release a book with details about my own life, and would have obsessed about every typo, missing period and the bad hair day I was having on the day my back cover photo was taken.

My healing journey was a long and tough one, filled with lots of reading, journaling and self-reflection...in between my scientific literature, diet and health books; I also read dozens of self-help books. You should have seen my nightstand!

While all of them were helpful, I was really excited when I found out that a book specific to those of us with Hashimoto's was coming out!

Stacey Robbins is a gifted, funny, honest and compassionate author. Reading her book is like speaking with an old friend who has been there and isn't afraid to tell you how it really is. Parts of the book left me in tears, others had me laughing. I had quite a few "Aha" moments, and saw myself in much of Stacey's writing. I found the book to be cathartic, empowering and uplifting at the same time.

Stacey bravely opens up her heart and life to show us how the circumstances in our life can affect our healing process, if we let them. She shares some of her own hardships and inspires us through showing how one can come out on top and how to go from victim to victor.

Stacey says: "This book is not a technical one, it's about shining the flashlight on the common issues and past experiences I've noted with thousands of Hashimoto's patients: Issues of perfectionism, fear and self-rejection -- past history of abuses and then perpetuating those abuses with a combination of over-attention to our complaints and yet an inattentiveness to our true needs."

I wish a book like "You're Not Crazy and You're Not Alone: Losing the Victim, Finding Your Sense of Humor and Learning to Love Yourself through Hashimoto's" was available earlier on my healing journey. I know that it will help you in yours!

Izabella Wentz, PharmD, FASCP
"Thyroid Pharmacist"
www.thyroidpharmacist.com

A Letter from a Friend

I don't have Hashimoto's. If I did, the first person I would call would be Stacey Robbins. I know Stacey would have answers. Maybe not *the answer* because that's not the way she works. She would have lots of answers and a whole lot more questions. She would also have gluten-free donuts sprinkled with what I love best about Stacey, her sweet compassion. Stacey offers cures – not necessarily just for Hashimoto's – for the soul. That's why I call her the soul whisperer.

Stacey's not a doctor. That doesn't discredit her from being one of the foremost experts on Hashimoto's. She's learned about the disease the hard way, by having it. Before knowing Stacey – and to know her is to know her because she doesn't hold any truths back – I had no idea Hashimoto's effected 200 million people, most of whom are my sisters. So even though I don't have Hashimoto's chances are I know someone who does.

In this book you will get the nitty and often gritty details of what it means to have a diagnosis of Hashimoto's. But don't be mistaken; Hashimoto's is merely the platform from which Stacey dives into your soul. Her message is for every one of us struggling with any kind of human condition. It's not gender specific. It's not age specific. You don't have to be on any one kind of a journey or another. You simply have to be, here and now, finding your way.

Stacey shares stories, insights and wisdoms that can heal whatever it is in us that is wounded. She has a way of turning your fear into your empowerment. She is the only person I know who can find the gift in Hashimoto's: The gift on not being able to lie about whom you are. The gift of not being able to cheat on yourself. The gift of not hiding in the dark any longer. I don't have Hashimoto's. If I did this book would make me feel for the first time that I'm not crazy and I'm not alone. I have Stacey. And now you do too.

She will open a door for you to a "whole" new kind of healing.

Tracy Panzarella
Certified Life/Health Coach

I'm Not a Doctor, but I'm Pretty Sure You're Not Crazy

I'm not a doctor
But I've been to plenty. More than my share. More than anybody's share.

I'm not a scientist.
I'm not even a wanna-be scientist. Though I *did* enjoy the periodic table of elements. Hated cutting open frogs and earthworms. The worms have 5 hearts you know, so you can cut them just about anywhere and they'll still live, which is kinda cool and kinda gross.

Cannot even believe I remember that. Quick, somebody put me on Jeopardy. "I'll take 'Random 8th Grade Science Facts' for $600, Alex.'"

The best secret I learned was to find the grungiest, earthiest boy to be your lab partner so he could do all of the dissecting, you could write the report, and you'd both get a good grade.

But I digress...

You're Not Crazy and You're Not Alone

Which will happen a lot in this book and you will, at the very least, be entertained. But you will be so much more than that. I promise.

I'm a student
And a sojourner
And a freedom-seeker.

I am a woman who was diagnosed with hypothyroidism in 1996 and Hashimoto's in 1999 and God-only-knows how long I had either or both before that. You would have thought Larry, Curly and Moe were running just about every medical office I went to those first few years, trying to figure out what was wrong with me – and being told forever and ever, amen that it was "anxiety." (See chapter called "Orange Cones." There's a section that deals with forgiveness.)

So, yeah. I've learned a few things in the almost 20 years of dealing with the symptoms and surprises of Hashimoto's and I want to share.

I've always loved show and tell. I love to write, and I love, love, love people.

I hate to see people suffer, which is why I want to offer any possible shortcut to those of you who are suffering. So that you don't have to learn the longer, harder way that I did. My heart is to provide some comfort from the fear of being sick, being tired, and being sick of being tired.

I'm here to tell you:

You're not crazy

I'm Not a Doctor but I'm Pretty Sure You're Not Crazy

And

You're not alone.

I also want you to know this:

Life is full of goodness

And

Health and healing are possible.

And I mean for *you*.

If you can get some of that from what I've learned – God, that just makes my heart a happier place to live.

I'm also a believer.

A believer in healing
And Love
And Love's ability to heal.

We are here for an unbelievable purpose.
That sometimes gets revealed to us through the painful process of a diagnosis.
And gets clarified through the unwieldy parts of life.

So, this book isn't going to be about telling you what to do (except sometimes) and it's not going to be about telling you who to go to (though, I will refer people in the back as resources so that I don't have to field 90,000 emails of who I went to and

You're Not Crazy and You're Not Alone

"Can I have her number?")

And this book isn't going to be your exhaustive resource on all things technical, mechanical, and anatomical about the dis-ease. Dear God, no.

I mean, I know a lot more about anatomy now, but I didn't always. Flashback 12 years ago when I was pregnant with my first son: there I was lying on the table, feet in the stirrups and legs spread to the far corners of the room.

(Did I mention that sometimes I'm going to give too much information?

Sorry.

By the way, sometimes, I'm going to give too much information.)

Anyway, where was I?

Oh yeah, legs spread on the table....

(Sorry, Mom.)

So, the doctor was down there saying something instructional about my girl bits and I said something like, "Oh, you mean my uvula?" The doctor looked up at me from between my legs to see if I was joking. My husband standing beside me looked at me in a slightly bemused way, knowing I wasn't.

He shook his head. "Hon, that's the dangly thing in the back of your throat."

I'm Not a Doctor but I'm Pretty Sure You're Not Crazy

I was like, "Really? That's what it's called? I thought that was the ulna."

Now the doctor raised her eyebrows and looked at Rocky. My husband, who knows me and who knows that I, despite being mostly wildly brilliant, can have my distinctly 'blonde' moments, closed his eyes and gave another little shake of his head, "That's part of your arm, babe."

"Really?" I stared back at him, not looking at him but more looking *through* him trying to find the word I was searching for, "I thought that was the vulva."

The doctor was in complete and utter disbelief. Rock answered in his usual straight man kind of way, "Now, *that's* what the doctor was talking about."

Dr. Beth turned to him, "Rocky, first of all, how do you know more about your wife's anatomy than she does? Second of all, please tell me she hasn't shared this information in public." My husband nodded, "I was paying attention in anatomy while she was drawing the word 'Love' and flowers around in her notebook."

I smiled. He was right.

He continued, "And yes, we had just about the same conversation with the new neighbor who introduced himself when we had just moved into the neighborhood. Stacey came out with a sore throat and we went through the whole thing, right in front of the poor guy, God, and everyone. And knowing my wife, she'll probably write about it somewhere for the entire world to see."

You're Not Crazy and You're Not Alone

And so, here it is.
For all the world to see.

Hello, world!

But I digress...

Point is, this book isn't heavy on science or anatomy. Yes, since that day on the examining table 12 years ago, I've learned significantly more than I knew then – I've had to – because when you're diagnosed with Hashimoto's and the people who are supposed to be experts don't give you sound advice, you have to start learning for yourself.

I've buried myself in health research, traveled all over the country for information, and spoken to people all over the globe for answers.

And while I am knowledgeable about many of the details and the physiology of Hashimoto's, this book is really more about shining a flashlight on some of the inner areas we deal with.

Those inner areas are about how we see ourselves and how we look at life.

Because if you think about it, Hashimoto's is an autoimmune disease.

That means that our body went into attack mode against itself. Our body is fighting against itself and treating our thyroid – which is a friend and gift we've been given – like it's an enemy.

I'm Not a Doctor but I'm Pretty Sure You're Not Crazy

That physical reality of attacking ourselves was already present for many of us as an emotional reality.

That's why I write it out that way: 'dis-ease' – with the hyphen in the middle. It's to remind myself, and all of us, that the part we are looking at is the dis-ease or un-ease we've had with ourselves. I believe, in most cases that the inner breakdown and lack of self-acceptance happened in our thought world and our belief system long before it ever showed up on our labs as a diagnosis.

After hearing the questions and issues of thousands of women with Hashimoto's, I've seen patterns in the way we think and in our life experiences. Common themes like self-hatred, perfectionism and self-rejection. That we struggle with guilt, fear and anxiety -- and that control and mistrust issues are driving us.

That there's been past abuse, which sets us up to reject ourselves. And we've used work-aholism and food issues to find some sense of control or comfort. Many of us have ended up having a repressed voice that has been trying to find its way to be truly expressed in the world.

Those things are so important, and dare I say, even possibly *more* so than what foods we eat and what supplements we take.

That's why these chapters may have a title like "Supplements" or "Exercise" but they're really not about that. I used those subjects as a jumping off point. Then, I allowed myself to go off on mystical tangents and story-telling for the sake of getting to the bigger points, all usually centered around issues of why we don't love our selves and the creative ways we come up with to sabotage our health.

You're Not Crazy and You're Not Alone

I really think you're going to love where it goes. And somewhere, in the reading of the tangents, you're going to see yourself in the story -- and something magical is going to be revealed for you.

I believe that with all my heart.

My aim is for us to see the deeper side of what we're dealing with so that we can be free. But I also want us to see the lighter side. We've been so sad and so serious for so long (and no, that bitter edge of sarcasm doesn't count as "happy".) God, we need to get off the stick that's been wedged up our ass and laugh a little more because life is funny when you start looking at it that way.

We need to start looking at it that way.

I want each of us to live as inspired, happy and healthy as we possibly can.

I promise, you're not alone in this: I've done tons of personal inner work. I've faced a lot of demons and found so many gifts in this process.

As I'm known for saying, "I may not be done, but I am different."

This process has been transformational for me.
And while I wouldn't have consciously raised my hand for Hashimoto's to be in my life, I can tell you that I'm sincerely grateful for what I have allowed it to produce in me.
My desire is to pass along whatever might be a good-wisdom, healing-thing, to you.

Disclaimer: In this book you will hear my stories, which include

I'm Not a Doctor but I'm Pretty Sure You're Not Crazy

swear words and frank talk about sex and religion. The one I really want to mention here is religion. In my stories you'll hear about my journey from Catholicism to Born-Again something-ism into Agnosticism with a few treasures of Buddhism, Humanism, Hinduism and Veganism (made you look) along the way. My ultimate landing point is that I believe God (The Divine, Source, The Great Spirit – whatever I may call God) is Love.

So, I just want to clear the deck before you read along and think I'm trying to evangelize you to some religion, because I'm not. I'm very clear in my intent: I'm trying to evangelize you to Love.

Loving yourself.
The Divine in you.
The Healer in you.

Part of why I wrote this book is that I imagined, what if someone I love were to come to me and tell me she had just been diagnosed with Hashimoto's or some other autoimmune thing, what would I say? What insights have I acquired that would benefit someone? This book is what I would share that I've learned as I've traveled this road and found valuable enough to pass along.

I want this information to serve you by showing you the possibilities that exist for your health and healing, inside and out.

Let me say this again, before anything else:

That you're not crazy
Despite what people think.
And you're not alone
Despite what you may feel.

You're Not Crazy and You're Not Alone

You're really not.

That would be the first thing I would tell my family
And my very best friends
And my close community.

Now that includes you.

Welcome to my circle. I'm really glad you're here.

So, there. That's my nutshell.
Pretty big nut, I know...

I hope you feel encouraged, inspired,
Slightly entertained, very curious,
A little disturbed...

But most of all, I really
Truly
From the bottom of my heart
Hope you feel
Deeply
And healing-ly
Loved.

-- Stacey Robbins October 2013, Newport Beach, California

Chapter 1

My Story: The Good, the Bad, the "Are You Kidding Me??" and the Grateful

Sometimes you're not sure where to start when you're writing your story. The questions come up of how much to highlight and whom you're going to hurt in the process of sharing – or worse, if by *not* sharing you're going to somehow hurt yourself once again, by not being true to your voice.

Life's never boring, is it?

This is my second pass at writing it out. You can tell how uncomfortable I am because I'm sitting in Susie's Cakes in Newport Beach, CA eating my weight in gluten-free banana pudding with real whipped cream.

Oh, and I have a gluten-free cupcake with espresso buttercream standing by, just in case of an emergency.

So, before I embark on "Take Two"...

You're Not Crazy and You're Not Alone

(the first take was 15 pages and over 6000 words. I really can't put either one of us through that. I figure, if I can't read it without wanting to jump off a cliff then, I shouldn't make you read it either)

...I want you to know something:

1. You are about to read some gnarly stuff.

It will go by quickly but you may see some of your gnarly stuff in my gnarly stuff. That's part of the point of me sharing. This whole life is one big game of 'connect the dots' – at a certain point, you put enough lines between the numbers and you get a clearer picture of what's going on. I believe that will start to happen for many who read this.

2. This gnarly stuff is not the whole picture.

These are significant events that got me into certain patterns of thinking and certain beliefs. So, these are sort of the high-lights of the lowlights, if that makes sense.

My life still had highlights, trust me. My life was not one long scene out of Oliver Twist.

I'm just not telling you all the good stuff from my life in this section (and there's been so much good, trust me) because I don't think it's the good stuff in my life that landed me with Hashimoto's, you know what I mean?

3. I learned valuable lessons from all of this.

So, even though the world around me was willing to let me be a victim and give me attention for some of the things that happened, there was something inside that never fully resonated with that. At some point, instead of seeing myself as a victim, I started to ask myself some important, and at times, uncomfortable questions:

  - *Why is this circumstance in my life?*

  - *Did I have any part in creating this?*

  - *Did my soul come here with a purpose and chose these pathways to gather lessons in order to inspire and teach others?*

  - *Or is this just the luck of the draw and I have the play this hand the best I know how?*

  - *Or something else?*

I find that in our world, we are either hyper-dumping responsibility, shame, and blame on ourselves or we are epidemically abdicating personal responsibility. I see overcompensating parents either trying to overcorrect an innocent child or over-assure a guilty one.

We see in politics, one party being demonized and another being canonized. We see celebrities given too much power for using their gifts and then, too little consequence when they have very ugly, human moments.
Whenever I see such extremes, I look for the lesson. When people have extreme reactions or take extreme positions, it's easy to miss the lesson that's hiding in there.

You're Not Crazy and You're Not Alone

<u>For example:</u> when the preacher is banging his fist on the pulpit screaming about how you're going to go to hell if you don't do this or that right, it would be easy to get swirled up in the fear of hell and miss the bigger lesson: <u>that Love is a better motivator than Fear is.</u>

So, whenever I see extremes that tempt to distract me, I ask myself, "What's the bigger point? And is it getting lost in all the fanfare?"

I had to ask those questions with Hashimoto's. I didn't want, on one extreme, to be treated terribly by the doctors, family members or friends who didn't understand -- but I also didn't want the other extreme of the world revolving around me. It was tempting to focus on the rejection that was on one end, and the over-attention on the other. Neither extreme were going to help me, serve me, or support my highest reason for being here.

I asked the questions, "What's the bigger point in having Hashimoto's? How can this serve me by helping me where I need to grow? What can I learn through having this?"

I want to learn the lessons that I need to learn in life. I want to share those lessons and have others share theirs. I want to heal and see others be healed.

I don't want to be the victim to the label of 'incurable' or anything else that comes with Hashimoto's. I don't want to be the poster child of the problem. I want to be a pioneer of the solution. That means I have to be willing to ask myself the hard questions in an atmosphere of love and grace:

> *- What is this about?*
> *- What part do I play in it?*
> *- Is the script already written or do I have the power to re-write the script?*
> *- If I have the power to write a new script going forward, does that mean I had the power to write the script that got me to this point?*

Big, huge, ginormous questions.

There's a lesson in all of it that has made my life richer so, I can't help but be grateful.

So, while I'm sharing the gnarly stuff, I'm sharing the stuff that moves me with gratitude. I can't stop myself. While I wouldn't have consciously written my script this way, I believe that all things can be used for my good.

It feels good and right to acknowledge that goodness.

4. **I love every one, and I mean EVERY one that I am writing about in this unconventionally written section of "My Story."**

I'm not blaming anyone, at least not anymore. I'm just identify-ing where stuff shows up. This is life, and here's a little secret: since we're connected, we can impact each other's lives with the stuff we do. To ignore that truth is to ignore the human and divine thread that connects us to each other. While I acknowl-edge the human failings, I want you also to know my love.

So, I'm breaking this up into three sections: **What Affected Me, Why I Share This, and What I'm Grateful For.**

What Affected Me:

My parents. Just as I'm in the powerful position of affecting my kids, all of our parents were in the powerful position of affecting us as children.

For as strong as my parents were in their strengths, they were as strong in their weaknesses. Their mix of passion and war made for a lot of marital stress and inconsistency in our home. Although they had tremendous gifts and taught me very good things that served me in life, they also had the dynamic where one was the lighter fluid and the other was the match. Not knowing when a fire would erupt left me walking on eggshells and feeling very insecure. I didn't trust that the good times would last and I didn't know when the bad times would come.

So, instead of playing with Barbie Dolls undistracted in the living room, I ended up with one eye on what I was doing and one on what my parents were up to. I was distracted by my concern for things heating up. I learned how to gauge the temperature of a conversation and tried to shift something from going in a scary direction. I felt an inordinate sense of responsibility for keeping myself safe and my family safe, as well.

Finally, there was an added pressure on me because I was expected to keep the damaging parts of our home life a secret. Those secrets made my intuition and sense of self-representation get stuck, maybe literally, in my throat.

The Good, the Bad, the "Are You Kidding Me??" & the Grateful

Why I Share This:

Because many Hashimoto's patients had either some kind of volatile or insecure childhood where they felt that they had to be in charge. They felt that way because they didn't feel they could trust those who were in charge to protect them. It's an overwhelming theme for women with Hashi's.

What I'm Grateful For:

I'm grateful for my parents for the totality of who they are. Truly. I'm not just saying that. But it was a process to get to this point. I heard the concept one day on a radio program that children choose their parents from the spirit-realm, before they are born. They do that because they know they will learn what they need to learn in order to do what they need to do in this world.

I had never heard that before and it intrigued me.

The idea that I 'chose' them as my parents, from what I call 'My Brave-Soul Place' was a liberating one to consider, because it allowed me to believe that my folks were perfect for what I needed to learn, in order to bring forth my purpose in the world. There was an interesting comfort in that thought.

I get to bring forward the obvious and overtly beautiful things my mom and dad taught me as well as the lessons from the unbeautiful ways they lived. I get to benefit from both, because I choose to.

And there's a side benefit, too: considering the idea that my kids chose me as their mom, released me from the perfectionism that threatens to overwhelm me. It helps me to see my imperfect places as 'perfect-for-them' places since my weaknesses will grow them, just as well as my strengths if they, too, will choose that. I am grateful to be able to share that empowering idea with them one day.

What Affected Me:

My Italian family members, who along with their big passionate love, noses and rear-ends, brought a lot of crazy. Crazy beliefs. Crazy superstitions. Crazy religion mixed with witchcraft. Crazy ideas of the role that men and women play. Crazy rejection and grudges if you broke the code (whatever that was). Crazy good cannoli. But still... *crazy*.

Why I Share This:

Because we create formulas from the people who are around us. We get impressions and messages on what it is to be a woman and what life is all about from the people who are in our close circle.

Plus, family dynamics can shape how we see "loyalty": who we're supposed to be loyal to, and who is supposed to be loyal to us, and what loyalty looks like. It isn't always healthy, especially when we're being asked to be loyal to a lie or to a secret. Family shapes us and those relational expectations can wreak havoc on us in later years.

The Good, the Bad, the "Are You Kidding Me??" & the Grateful

What I'm Grateful For:

I'm grateful for all the characters and caricatures – but I'm also grateful to have learned this: just because a family member says something, doesn't mean it's true.

Because I know how crappy it felt when I was rejected by my family when I stood for my truth, I now get to empower my children to consider what I say and to measure it against their truth rather than their loyalty to me. I tell my kids: be loyal to the truth, be committed to people.

What Affected Me:

The drug dealer who apparently respected that I wouldn't take the freebie drugs he was offering around to the neighborhood kids. So, on Halloween night, when I was 12 years old, he climbed into my bedroom window and raped me while my parents were in the next room. He proceeded to do that for months and threatened that he'd hurt my sisters, if I told anyone. I became an expert secret-keeper.

Why I Share This:

Many Hashi's women were abused in some way. Many were told they had to keep it a secret. When secrets get swallowed, where do they go? What kind of stress do they cause? Are they part of the Hashimoto's profile? Well, I see the common thread of abuse and a lack of self-representation in this dis-ease.

You're Not Crazy and You're Not Alone

What I'm Grateful For:

I am grateful because I learned that you can go through something that is victimizing and still have the power to choose whether or not you're going to become a victim for life.

What Affected Me:

The adult family member who I reached out to and told about the rapes and asked for his help: instead of helping, he ended up molesting me, too.

Why I Share This:

I rarely ever share this, but I am in this book for this reason: abuse often repeats itself in the Hashimoto's personality and history. It is very common to hear of someone being raped more than once or having a variety of abuses in her lifetime. If this happened to you, I want you to know, you're not crazy and you're not alone.

I am keenly aware that, for some of you reading this, this is the first time you ever heard that you are not alone in this. I'm sending you peace and comfort to your heart right now.

What I'm Grateful For:

I am grateful for forgiveness that is as great as the offense. When you have come, vulnerable and in need, to a person whom you trust and then, that person, instead of protecting you, violates you – it requires a different level of forgiveness than if a stranger were to have hurt you. I also learned that being forgiving has a lot *of power in unhinging <u>you</u> from the event and allows you to live in forward motion.*

And I learned that a child's trust is sacred. Handle it with care.

What Affected Me:

The religious people who brought a mixed message that a punishing God is a loving God. That theology really resonated with the mixed message in my home. When you hear, "I'll punish you because I love you" from an angry parent or, "I'll send you to hell because I love you" from an angry God, that doesn't generate a trusting devotion. It generates a fear and a formulaic, inorganic relationship. When that happens, you're not able to live your life and your unique purpose, because you are trying to figure out how to keep the God of the Universe happy so that you can avoid his wrath.

Beside all that, as a child, I was just trying to figure out how all this bad stuff could happen and still maintain my hope and belief in a God who made me and loved me. That mixed message messed with my head. Deeply.

Why I Share This:

When we have unhealthy definitions of what Love is, we will find other places and relationships to play out our messed up understandings of Love.

For me, and for many with Hashi's, I have heard their frustration because they sincerely want to be in a loving relationship with a loving God, but they're just terrified. It's one thing to have a screwed up relationship with a parent or spouse, but to have a messed up perception of God can shape your whole understanding of who you are and why you're here. It's a big deal and it can cause a lot of stress. Stress is not a friend to your thyroid.

What I'm Grateful For:

I am grateful that the same people who taught me crazy theology also taught me to seek God and to seek Truth. As a result of following that bit of golden advice, I have found a greater understanding of God. Along with that, I have a greater peace with the truth that I've found, than the truth I was taught.

Anyone who teaches you a bigger truth, regardless of how they're living, has given you a gift that will bring you freedom.

What Affected Me:

The two car accidents that happened in one year, right before I was diagnosed with Hypothyroidism – and the courts that didn't compensate me for them. I woke up in pain and lived all day in pain until I went to bed in pain. That lasted about two years. When pain lasts that long, you forget what it feels like to feel normal.

Why I Share This:

If I had a dollar for every Hashi's person who told me that they were diagnosed after either whiplash from a sport injury or a car accident, I could get a massage every day this year. I don't want to miss addressing this common occurrence as a possible trigger for Hashimoto's.

What I'm Grateful For:

I am grateful that I wasn't fully compensated for my injuries. Had I won those cases with big bucks (I won both cases, just not with big bucks) I may have been indoctrinated with the idea that injury = compensation and reverted to that low vibrational formula for the rest of my life. I may have been so content being the rewarded victim that I never pursued the bigger questions I've considered.

And I learned a valuable lesson from my lawyer: that about 75% of people, injured in an accident, begin to heal when the court case is done. I concluded that it must take a lot of energy to have to represent how victimized and injured we are and that we probably arrest our healing for the sake of having to represent our pain. So, basically, we stay hurt to prove how badly we were hurt. That lesson was a tremendous gift to me. Don't want to live that way. No bueno.

What Affected Me:

My husband's hidden issue with pornography that probably started when he was a teen, to anesthetize him from the pain of his mom dying when he was young. I discovered his issue a few months after we were married. It brought into our marriage rejection, pain, and more secrets. More double-life kind of living. It further perpetuated the story I had, that I wasn't worth loving.

You're Not Crazy and You're Not Alone

Why I Share This:

It's important for me to see the patterns that we play out. We have a belief that we're reject-able and unworthy of love and then, we pick someone who is rejecting of us and makes us feel unworthy. There are two valuable things in that:

1. Seeing where our patterns play out.
2. Getting off the thing of blaming the other person for being the way they are.

We have to look at what belief we brought to the table that had us choose this person with these issues. Seeing the truth will free us. That's an uncomfortably good thing to see.

What I'm Grateful For:

I am grateful that I got a chance to face my own lust – a lust to be in control, which was my kickback response to fear. I'm grateful that I started looking at myself and what my issues were. Pain is never wasted when you use it to help you grow.

I'm grateful for the fact that my husband walked away from pornography at year seven of our marriage and that I was 270 lbs., and not 135 lbs. Because had I been skinny and darling instead of ginormous and cranky, I would have gotten the message that his faithfulness was tied to me being 'good enough'. That would have made me the manager of his fidelity and given me a power I should never have. But because he left his vice during the time I was my heaviest, I got the powerful message that you don't have to be perfect in order to be loved.

The Good, the Bad, the "Are You Kidding Me??" & the Grateful

What Affected Me:

The doctors who misdiagnosed me, mistreated me, and misinformed me. Who told me it was all in my head... who told me that I could just take a pill and feel better, and scooted me out of their offices. Especially that one doctor who told me I was wasting his time and why did I insist on interrupting his lunch with my imaginary problems. *Sigh.*

Why I Share This:

It's important for women who have Hashi's to hear this. Why? Because most of us received this message growing up:

"Trust your leaders/doctors/authority figures."

And that's good except for this: it puts the power, always, someplace else.

Had we been taught to also honor our intuition and inner knowing, we would have been equipped to have power as well. But so many of us were taught to squash our power because we were taught to ignore our inner truth in order to keep a family secret or because our truth would have caused too many problems for others.

I can't tell you how many women with Hashi's enter the doctor's office vulnerable to share their symptoms and wanting to respect their doctor, yet, because these women don't allow themselves to listen to that little voice that said, "This is not honoring" when their doctor is discounting them, they end up very hurt. And worse, they end up following treatments that may be damaging and off-course for them.

I want those women to know that they are not crazy and they are so not alone.

What I'm Grateful For:

I am grateful when doctors get dethroned as 'all-knowing gods' and are put in the category of simply 'human.' It takes the pressure off of them to know what they don't know and it shares the onus with us, their patients. We need to be empowered to own our health journey with responsibility and knowledge – as well as find trustworthy doctors who will partner with us in the journey.

I'm grateful for the chance to see all of those doctors as gifts to me, whether they had the right answer or not. The ones who did, led me toward health, the ones who didn't also led me toward health by being an Orange Cone. An Orange Cone doesn't give you the answer, it tells you to "Go around!" which I learned to do and, as a result, I found other resources who helped me and beautiful wisdoms in unexpected places.

What Affected Me:

Those friends and family members and co-workers over the years who didn't understand, were rude, presumptuous, and judgmental of me not feeling well...*again.* That they were disappointed in me not living up to their dreams of what they thought I should be. They bailed on me when I needed someone the most and could have used an ounce of compassion instead of a pound of disdain.

The Good, the Bad, the "Are You Kidding Me??" & the Grateful

Why I Share This:

Because there's a woman who's out there feeling crazy for how hurt she feels because of her family. She's feeling like she let everyone down and instead of that family member or friend putting a comforting arm around her, they crossed their arms and stood back and judged. It compounds the pain when you are feeling so sick on the inside and then so unsupported on the outside.

What I'm Grateful For:

I am grateful that I learned to be able to trust my own voice, despite their voices of criticism in my head. I'm enormously grateful for the day I realized that their voice was just an external representation of my internal critic, and that if I would stop judging myself so harshly, I would find that oft times, they would stop, too. That was a great lesson to me – to look beyond the person's face to the person's reflection and ask myself: what are they reflecting that lives in me? I learned the greatest pathway to loving someone who was challenging to me, was to love that part of me that was challenging to me.

So, that's my story, or at least the challenging bits that led up to my Hashimoto's diagnosis.

Hard things have happened: insecure home life, sexual abuses outside of the home, eating disorders, harsh religious beliefs, car accidents, absent partners, judgmental friends and family, and discompassionate doctors....

These are the common threads I've found in Hashimoto's as I've been in community with thousands of women around the world:

That we overwork ourselves and overburden ourselves with responsibility.

That we tend to focus on our weaknesses rather than our strengths and give ourselves a ridiculously hard time.

That we tend to overthink about things, and yet under-care for our body and spirit.

That we get ourselves into toxic relationships that make us feel like crap, and then try to control the relationship and get that toxic person to love us.

That we're amazing. Deep thinking, hard-working, high-ethic people who care profoundly for others and for life, and truly want to make a difference here.

That we are dream-makers and idea people. Powerful and agents of change in the world. We are often speakers, writers, musicians and other types of expressively, creative people – despite, or because of, this little butterfly-shaped gland at the base of our throat, near our voice box, that seems to be having a hard time getting along in this world.

My heart for us is to heal. And that whatever story we came in with that isn't empowering, we would shift to empowering. And whatever part we came in with that isn't inspiring, we would shift to inspiring. And whatever part we came in with that isn't love, we would shift to the greatest healing and freeing force there is: Love.

I'm Not a Doctor but I'm Pretty Sure You're Not Crazy

That our story we came in with would end up being a great Love story. One that we live with. And lead with. And leave with.

That through our Hashimoto's journey,
ours would be a Legacy of Love in the world.

Chapter 2

Fettuccine Alfredo, Donut Holes, and Other Crimes of Passion

If I were told that I had only one final meal to eat before I went to that great Big Buffet in the sky, it would probably be a buttery, extra-creamy, four-cheese Fettuccine Alfredo (with extra Pecorino Romano on top, please) and a package of chocolate, glazed donut holes from Entenmann's Bakery.

And then, I would die a happy woman, entering the pearly gates in a state of food-orgasmic bliss.

Only one problem: If you eat that way with Hashimoto's and it's NOT your last meal, you'll kinda wish it were.

Oh, how I remember that fateful day...

(Warning: *way* TMI coming soon.)

...consuming the unbelievable melt-in-your-mouth fettuccine pasta my aunt had made by hand. She let them swim in a lake of the creamiest, dreamiest, cheesiest Alfredo sauce a person could ever make.

I shlurped.
I cooed.
I ooh-ed
and I mmmm-ed
to the point that it was probably embarrassing, but I really didn't care.

I'm pretty sure I said "OhmyGOD!!!" more than a Southern Baptist preacher or a 42nd Street prostitute (and possibly even more than a Southern Baptist preacher *with* a 42nd Street prostitute). I couldn't help myself. I was too busy with the fettuccine love affair I had going.

Just an aside: this was *before* I had the complete wake-up call of what dairy did to me, and it was kind of in the *middle* of the wake-up call of what gluten did to me.

It was when I still believed you could have 'just a little', 'every so often' which would conveniently turn into, 'just between my birthday in November and all the way through Christmas to New Year's Eve.' I can't remember how many times on New Year's Day, I laid on the couch, half-dead, trying to figure out which truck had just hit me. It's hard to write your New Year's resolutions when all you want to do is crawl into a hole and die.

On this auspicious day, the Fettuccine Alfredo *became* my wake up call of what gluten and dairy did to me.

Yes. See, here's how it goes: when you put together gluten from the pasta, and the dairy from the OhmyGOD!!! sauce, you essentially have the formula for weapons of mass destruction.

Right there.
In the petri dish
Otherwise known as 'my stomach.'

OhmyGOD!!! it tasted so good...

I felt the first gurgle. But I kept on eating.
I felt the rumbles. But I had another round.

Somewhere around my second bowl of fork-twirling delight, it happened.

My eyes opened wide. My butt-clenched tight. I swallowed hard, and prayed softly for mercy. I practically knocked over my folding chair as I pushed back from the table, my napkin falling from my lap. I managed to eek out a pinched, "Bathroom?? UPstairs??!!!" to my hostess, while sweat started beading over my lip.

Without even waiting for an answer, I ran to the staircase while my 14 Italian relatives stared at me. I held the wooden banister with my left hand and tried, desperately, to unbutton my pants with my right while I tripped up the steps and got to the bathroom with barely a moment to spare. Slapping the unfamiliar wall for the switch, I flipped on the light and groaned.

No fan.

No noise.

You're Not Crazy and You're Not Alone

No nothing.

Not a sound to cover up the detonations of weapons of mass destruction that were about to happen.

There was just an open window.
Over the tub.
Right above the open slider door where everyone was sitting below eating dinner.

I sat on the potty trying to not die.

And trying to not ruin the meal of every. single. person eating the best Fettuccine Alfredo in the world at the table, right underneath the bathroom.

If I had been 9 years-old, I might have started humming, or even singing. If I were 13, I may have turned on the sink or flushed the toilet a million times.

But I was 38 and couldn't find a solution in my head because I was too busy pooping my brains out and groaning, "OhMyGODDD!!!" for a completely different reason than I had just minutes before.

Now, I was praying.

Praying to not die.
Praying for the pain and suffering to end.
Praying for everyone to go instantly deaf.
And whatever it's called when you want people to not be able to smell, either.

Fettuccine Alfredo, Donut Holes, and Other Crimes of Passion

All of this 'fun' and 'excitement',

Just because I didn't want to give up certain foods.

Because 'food' was my culture.
'Food' was my life.
'Food' made me feel alive. Like I was living 'the good life.'
'Food' made me *happy*.

(Note: sitting on the toilet that day. Weapons of mass destruction. Trying to not die. Not feeling alive. Not living the good life. Definitely NOT *happy*.)

Food...
It's a tricky one.

Honestly, it's a button-pushing topic for many of us with an auto-immune thing.

I remember in the beginning of being sick almost 20 years ago and then, the diagnoses a few years later. I was looking for a miracle:

"God, YOU do it!"

And while I certainly believe in the spiritual component to the whole thing and that reaching out to the Divine is a great, healing thing, I wasn't getting all the results I wanted.

Then, I switched to, "Doctors, YOU (and your synthetic meds) do it!"

You're Not Crazy and You're Not Alone

There are good doctors out there, and they helped me some. I'm grateful for the good they bring to the table but I wasn't getting all the help I needed.

Next, I found the natural route and I was like, "Supplements, acupuncture, Reiki, Jin Shin, NAET, and on and on and on: YOU do it!"

Luh-OVE natural remedies. I'm a believer. But after a scrillion expensive tests and gobs of supplements, I still wasn't where I wanted to be.

All the while messages were coming to me:

Change your lifestyle.
Change your relationships.
Change your rest.
Change your food.

Essentially: Stacey, YOU do it.

I couldn't deflect responsibility onto anything else or make anyone else my Obi Wan. I had to look at my to-do list and see what I needed to do, that no one else could do for me.

Honestly, I think I wanted to do anything but change my food.

Being raised in an Italian family with my mom as an amazing cook and my grandmother as an amazing baker meant I grew up having an unbelievable foodie experience. My great aunts would churn homemade sausages and grow the peppers that they'd roast over the fire to put in jars of olive oil for the antipasto. My great-grandmothers would wake up at 3 a.m. just to make the bread, pluck the chickens, and fry up the chicken livers for the dog.

Even the dog was a gourmand.

This was my food experience.

Food was my life, my culture, my sense of belonging, my holidays, my pride, my liberty... my *identity*.

It was attached to my sense of fun when I went out with my friends, because 'fun' meant I could eat and drink any way I wanted.

And food was attached to my dreams of the future:

"When I go to Italy, I will eat my way through Amalfi and all the way down to Sicily."

How does one go to Italy and NOT eat the pasta?
Is life even worth living if you can't go to Italy and drink the wine and eat the bread???

It has been SUCH a process of surrender. For me to redefine the 'Life of My Dreams' as a life where I eat and drink whatever I want -- to 'The Life of My Dreams' meaning that I feel good again.

Trust me, I really wanted a pill to make it better. And if you told me that I could have slept long enough to heal myself of this thing, I would have gladly gone into hibernation.

So, why do I share this? Because I understand how it's more than letting go of gluten and dairy, corn and eggs, soy and night-shades and grains. It's about letting go of all the associations we make with food.

I did all those other things on the list – I took care of my relation-ships, rest, supplements, meds, lifestyles, etc… They're all valu-able and essential, but none of them are a substitute for what only the food changes can provide.

Myalgias went away, weight was lost, depression lifted, deeper sleep came, clarity of thinking returned, and internal order resur-faced. I had no idea that cake was making me bitchy and that raw veggies made me want to have sex again. Who knew?

- I didn't know that my palpitations and racing heart were coming from food.
- That the anxiety I was feeling was coming from what I ate.
- That the tingling in my toes was from my menu choices.
- That the heavy chest and labored breathing were from all I had consumed.

I had no idea the powerful role that food plays in our health… until I removed certain foods.

Before that, it was all theory and other peoples' opinions, which I staunchly disagreed with. I firmly believed that anyone who was telling me to eliminate certain foods was being *extreme*.

So, please know, if you're new to this whole thing or been dealing with Hashi's for a long time and have been unwilling to dive into the deep water of food changes – I understand.

Fettuccine Alfredo, Donut Holes, and Other Crimes of Passion

When you hear me, or other folks with Hashi's beating the drum about making some food changes, it's not because anyone's trying to ruin your fun or create some cultic thinking. It's because many of us have traveled the long journey of trying to change everything BUT our food, and we want to short cut you to one of the quickest ways you can start feeling better.

My advice is this: really consider looking at a food elimination program. I personally love AIP (Autoimmune Paleo Protocol) but there are many other ways: Weston A. Price, Gerson Therapy, SCD (Specific Carbohydrate Diet), The Plan by Lyn Genet and on and on...

For me, I was a vegetarian for the longest time. I was at my highest weight – probably because I was a 'Fettuccine Alfredo' kind of vegetarian with an undiagnosed thyroid issue and not an 'eat a big, green leafy salad' kind of vegetarian. One day, I went to a sassy, Italian Naturopath who said, "You have to eat meat. You're anemic; you have high triglycerides, high cholesterol and low thyroid. You need meat."

Oh God, I cried. I started with fish. The teeniest, tiniest bits of white fish, that we had to go to a restaurant for because I couldn't look at it or touch it, let alone cook it. I ate it with a toothpick instead of a fork, literally crying over the plate. I called my mother after my first serving of fish in over 10 years, looking for some compassion. She dryly said, "Did all of your organs get up and give you a standing ovation?"

Gee, thanks, Mom.

After about four days of that, I thought I was going to grow gills.

You're Not Crazy and You're Not Alone

I switched to a restaurant that would make me the teeniest, tiniest, bits of chicken that I ate with the tip of a toothpick.

A month later my triglycerides were normal, I stopped being anemic, I lost weight and my cholesterol went down.

A year later, I ate my first hamburger and I've never looked back.

Because the proof was in the pudding. Or in my case, the meat.

Which makes me think of 'meat pudding' which is really gross.

Sorry.

(P.S. for those of you who are vegetarians, vegans, raw vegans, pescatarians… this is not a book about pushing meat on you, this is my journey. I wanted to be a vegetarian, my body was proving that it did better with meat. If you've found a way to optimize your health with your no-meat plan, please hear me, you have my respect and my support.)

I've added some other great habits over the years: raw juicing, whole food supplements, spirulina and other things. It was a steady progression to shift my food choices from what they were, then, to what they are today.

The people who don't want to hurt your feelings will tell you to *limit* toxic foods. I know this news will help you so, I'm going to shoot straight: you can't limit a poison and have it be good for you.

Figure out what foods are toxic to you and eliminate them. Once your gut heals enough, you can sometimes reintroduce those eliminated foods back into your life – on an occasional basis or permanently. Anything is possible. But for now, a toxic food is a toxic food. I'm not sure how having a little bit of poison in your system makes it less a poison. It doesn't.

Eggs made me cry. I loved them and ate them every day. But still, despite my affection and deep devotion to them, they made me cry. Then, I learned that it was my sensitivity to something in the eggs and I decided to eat them every few days instead of every day.

I thought that was "reasonable."

So, I cried every few days instead. (I'm rolling my eyes right now.)

And then, I was like, "Wow. I wouldn't have to cry *any* days if I just stopped eating the eggs for a while..."

So, I did. And I stopped crying. Wow. Amazing how that happens. You take an offending food away and lo and behold, your body stops being offended! And now, months later, I can have eggs every so often and I don't even cry one, little bit.

Gone are the weapons of mass destruction.

Gone are the holidays and birthdays that start off great and then, I "treat" myself (to poison, because you know, it's my birthday and I deserve to poison myself...Huh?) and end up feeling like crap.

Gone are the erratic emotional rollercoasters that come from the chemical reaction that food makes in our system.

You're Not Crazy and You're Not Alone

Gone are the days when I make a special event, more important than *me*.

Or my health.
Or my presence to my family.
Or my sense of wellness.
Or my future.

I really want your journey to feeling better to be shorter than mine has been so, the encouragement and experience I want to offer is this: face the food issues head-on.

It's not a sacrifice, when you realize your worth.

It's an investment in the most important person in your life:

You.

"The food you eat can either be the safest and most powerful form of medicine or the slowest form of poison." Ann Wigmore

Chapter 3

Oh, My Mother Thinks I'm Special (But I Just Feel Like a Freak)

So, you're a unique bird, right?

Me, too.

How many of our moms said, "There's no one like you in *all* the world?"

And it's true. There isn't.

And yet, when we end up with Hashimoto's, we can tend to feel a sense of, "Yeah, there's not one. single. person like me in all the world. I'm alone. A freak and alone."

We start noticing that we can't eat the things our husband's can. We can't go the places our friends can go. We can't do the things our kids can do.

We feel unique, but not in a good way.

We're all gonna have that moment when we say, "Man, everyone else can have this but I can't."

You're Not Crazy and You're Not Alone

And then, we hear our mother's voice saying to us in our head, "If everyone were going to jump off the Brooklyn Bridge, would you?"

To which I would answer, "No. But I'd really like to eat bacon without gaining 12 lbs or eat grilled onions without having to clear the house from the wild toot-fest and writhing stomach pains that follow and..."

We all have something.

We're all unique.

Some people say, "Oh, if you have Hashimoto's, don't eat goitrogens unless they're cooked!"

To which I say, "I can't eat goitrogens, even when they're cooked, unless I want to gain 3 pounds and my fingers start to swell like they belong on the Michelin Tire Man."

Oh, but I love them! Give me steamed broccoli with garlic and olive oil, or a plate of mashed cauliflower with tons of garlic and I'm in h-e-a-v-e-n.

Yeah. But I'll pay for it.

It's kind of weird to be willing to gain three pounds for eating a vegetable.

It's funny how my "cheat" foods are broccoli, rice, eggs, dairy and hot sauce. I remember when my "cheat foods" were a pan of brownies or a dish of pecan pie, a la mode.

Oh, My Mother Thinks I'm Special (But I Just Feel Like a Freak)

It's a different time.

I get it.

And it's all good. Because I don't call my foods 'limited', I call them 'focused.'

It helps my mindset and for me see the abundance in my choices and that they're *for* me. Nothing's being kept *from* me. I can choose to eat anything. It's just that some things are going to make me feel like shit and some are not. I choose to *focus* my foods on what makes me feel good.

(Well, most of the time, anyway...)

I remember when I was considering doing a raw food diet. I kept hearing it call to me but it was a concept that was so far away from the 'cook everything to death' candida protocol I had been doing for months before.

The candida protocol was good and valuable and I felt that Wisdom had led me to it, but I was feeling drawn another way. The *raw* way. One of my practitioners was trying to dissuade me, "Oh Stacey! You can't do that! Raw foods are going to make you bloat and give you gas and you're going to feel just terrible!"

Something inside me just said, "Go for it."

And I did! Big arugula salads and TONS of raw onions -- God, I love raw onions, can't eat them cooked without having major stomach issues, but man, I can eat them raw – no problem! Plus there's lots of great Quercetin in them! Then, I added strawberries, raw cheddar, with a scant few raw sliced almonds, some cooked chicken or salmon....and God, I swear, I heard the angels sing.

All those overcooked foods, that I had been eating before made me bloated. All of them made my fingers swell. The raw foods made me feel alive, my tummy got flat, and I was satisfied.

My friends were mystified. My naturopath was not. Dr. Barrett shrugged her shoulders and said, "Well, sounds like you have an enzymatic issue. Every food has its own enzyme to break it down. When it's cooked, it has less of its own enzyme and has to use the enzymes in your body to break the food down. Raw foods have more of the enzymes still in tact and require less from your body. Sounds like raw veggies and cooked meats work for you. Go for it."

I felt like I had won the lottery. Because once you figure what works out for uniquely you and you feel good, you stop worrying about all the food trends and agendas that people have for you to do their program. You stop worrying about who says what you're doing shouldn't work and why.

And trust me, I hold loosely to what works for me. I realize that as my body heals, my hormones change, as I age, or travel or whatever, that things may need to be adjusted. I just need to keep listening for Wisdom and what works best for my body.

And I don't need everyone else to understand in order for me to honor my uniqueness.

I also don't expect everyone to bow to it either.

Oh, My Mother Thinks I'm Special (But I Just Feel Like a Freak)

I am not the center of the universe and everything doesn't revolve around me. When I go out to dinner with friends, I order my food, but I don't make what I'm eating the center of the conversation (anymore). I'm there to be with friends and we're all part of the community.

I don't need my attention in life to come to me because I happen to order my meals like Sally from When Harry Met Sally (which I do – minus the public orgasm -- which would be entertaining the first few times...but after that, not so much.)

My food explanations might be interesting, for the moment, but at some point, healthy people want to talk about something other than why you have to ask the waiter if there's soy sauce in that stir fry, because, "No, soy sauce isn't gluten-free..."

Your friends will say, "Oh really?"

"Yes, really," you will say, "and let me tell you the molecular reasoning behind 'why'..."

People are going to stop asking you out.

Just because you have food sensitivities, doesn't mean you have to turn into the science teacher and the gathering into a class on biogenetics.

(Snore.)

Anyway, back to the subject at hand. (What were we talking about again?)

You're Not Crazy and You're Not Alone

I really wish I were one of *those* people – you know -- the folks who are like my husband: who can go anywhere, eat anything, sleep in any bed, and poop in any bathroom. The one who's *easy.*

Yeah…That's. Not. Me.

Like my husband has been known to say, "You're complicated, but you're worth it."

To which I say, "Thank you."

And then, I think, *Heyyyy, wait a minute…*

I've finally (mostly) stopped feeling guilty for being the complicated one.

(Which by the way, I now use the word 'complex' -- it sounds more generous – sort of like the universe is complex but it's not complicated. It makes me feel more expansive and less pain-in-the-assive.)

I need to take care of me in my uniqueness, and you need to take care of you in yours.

If my taking care of me in any way, means you have to stop taking care of you, then our balance is off. We're each responsible for our own stuff. No one is the martyr here and no one is more important than the other.

Now, I'm just going to pause here, because I know that so many women are living with a partner who just. doesn't. get it. I KNOW! Oh, God. Yes, we will be talking about that in the future. It may have to be its own separate book. Sigh.

So, right now you may be feeling like I'm picking on the wrong person, here. Right?

No. I'm not picking on you. *You're* the one in this conversation. If your partner were reading this book right now, I would say to him, "Stop being such a all-fired weenie!" (I really wanted to use another word beside 'weenie' but I showed unbelievable restraint. I hope you're proud of me.)

"This woman is going through hell. Her life is sprained, not broken. Don't be deluded into thinking that, just because she's not lying in a hospital bed with a cast all over her doesn't mean she's not fighting for her life right now.

Just because she can still function in some ways doesn't mean that her system isn't under extreme duress.

It is.

Your thyroid controls EVERYTHING in your body. And having it be out of whack affects every cell in the body. You think that something small getting hit doesn't throw your system down? Let's do a little experiment on you getting hit between the legs and let me know how that doesn't bring you to your knees...

She needs your help. Your compassion. Your research. Your understanding. You to be there when she's at the doctor's, trying to sort stuff out with all this brain fog she's got. She needs you to look into what's going on so that you can get your big, ripe head out of your ass and be part of the solution instead of part of the problem."

So, see...yeah. That's what I would say. But here's the thing: it's likely *you*, who have Hashimoto's, who are reading this book and it's not your spouse. Which reminds me of when I used to say to my counselor, "Hey! That's great information. Can you go tell it to my husband? He's the one who really needs to hear this!" And she'd say, "I can only treat the person in front of me, who is present, and willing to be treated."

You're reading the book so, we're working *your* stuff out. Make sense?

Until the other people in your life are inspired to change, they're not going to. So, what are you going to do in the meantime? You're going to address your shit so that you're not tripping yourself through this marathon called *Life*. You've got to start being your own best friend. Waiting for someone else to take action, who isn't enlightened about what to do, is setting you up to be a victim to them.

That was a huge tangent and I totally digressed.
And it was totally worth it.

You okay over there?

The point is this: I want to help us to lose the victim we have in us. I want to empower us to address what we need to address within. We can't spend our life waiting to take care of us because someone else isn't getting it.

Chronic victimhood, which can sometimes be the bedfellow to

chronic dis-ease, is going to lead to resentment on both sides of a relationship. We have times where someone may need more than another person in another season, yes. But we're here by choice, and that means powerfully choosing not to let your diagnosis become the all-consuming, never-ending focus of the relationship.

And besides, we all have something we're dealing with: for you it might be crooked toes that make you walk funny, for me, it's Hashimoto's. We're all special.

Which makes me think of Dash from The Incredibles who said, "If everyone's special, then nobody's special."

I think that's funny because it kind of equalizes us and puts us all on level ground. But truthfully, I do believe we're all uniquely special – no one in the world like us.

We're here for a unique purpose and some of us have some unique idiosyncrasies and sensitivities on this side of eternity. Pay attention to them, take care of them, honor them where you can, and kill them when they don't serve you. That's fine. It's all good. Let your freak flag fly.

Just don't wave it in my face.

As my mother would say,

"Be careful! There are people around you!

You could poke an eye out with that thing."

Chapter 4

Orange Cones and Lessons in Forgiveness

I had lost count of how many doctor's appointments I had been to.

This one was my main guy, my primary care physician. A friend had referred him and raved so, I had jumped on board with him about a month before my entire life fell apart that Spring of 1995.

My grandmother had just passed. My father (her son) at a mere 49 years-old was dying, and I had just been hit in the first of two car accidents.

Oh, and I was separated from my husband.

After six hard years of dealing with a 'compulsive habit' (we didn't use the word 'addiction') that my husband didn't want to face, I finally said, "Enough. I don't want to divorce you. I just need some space to heal."

If there were ever a perfect storm of events to help a body to crash and burn, this was probably it.

So, the doctors visits that started with complaints of stomach aches from stress, that turned into pain from accidents, and then sickness coming from what I thought was grief upon grief.

This doctor, Dr. Tom, we'll call him, never knew me in all my healthy years or wellness check-ups where I'd just breeze in, hop up on the table and be told, "You're as healthy as a horse." Nope. I pretty much met him and then, soon after, my life fell to pieces like shards of shattered glass in front of him.

He seemed affable enough in the beginning, and was even concerned. Though, he was doling out drugs in a pretty casual manner. By the end of seven months, I had been on antibiotics seven times for chronic sinus infections and eight other prescriptions to deal with everything from back pain from the car accidents, to anti-depressants, to cholesterol lowering drugs, to weight loss meds.

Ah yes, the days of Fen-Phen ...

Dr. Tom put me on double the dose for the unusual, unexplained weight gain I was experiencing. It was hard for me to understand how I was gaining so much weight, so quickly, since I didn't feel a bit of hunger. I still had a personal trainer and was writing down every bite of food.

The Fen-Phen was known for amping people up. That extra 'amp' only fed the anxiety that was a new and increasing in my life. My heart racing out of my chest was a phenomenon I'd never had before.

Rocky usually came with me to these doctor visits. We had shared most of our flexible self-employed musician's life together and had a deeply connected bond. But, because I was so hurt by his destructive choices, I was trying life solo in an attempt to heal from our marriage stuff.

I was alone.

My vulnerability was even greater that day with Dr. Tom.

I walked in to his office asking to be seen since I knew I had another sinus infection. Plus, I was still having pain from a half hour after I awakened every morning until I went to sleep crying at night. It was intense. I worked 80-90 hours a week, singing and piano performances as well as teaching … I didn't have time for this.

How ironic, because neither did Dr. Tom.

Instead of a compassionate and curious, "Why is this happening, Stacey? Oh, wait! I'm a doctor, let me investigate…" I got a curt and condescending response from him that day. He seemed jittery, almost like he was jacked up on something, though, I've never been good at telling two things: when people are on drugs and when women have had boob jobs. I just am clueless about both. In retrospect, Dr. Tom was clearly on something.

Maybe 'being mean' is a drug.

He put his arm around my shoulder in a strong, uncomforting way one might lead a child outside to be disciplined. He moved me out of the office and through the waiting room until we were standing near the front door.

He talked to me in a sick whisper and a forced smile on his face the whole time, "Why do you *insist* on taking my lunch time away from me? There is nothing wrong with you." Proving that you can actually hiss *and* have a smile on your face, "This is all psychological ... in your *head*, Stacey. So, why don't you go home, young lady, and stop wasting my time. How many times are you going to take my lunch time away from me?" He gave me a little shove onto the sidewalk with those last words.

I waited until I was in the car, locked inside, before I burst into tears.

Alone.

No husband to be with me.
No father to understand.
No doctor to help me.

Alone.

I laid my head down on the steering wheel. I squeezed my eyes tight just trying to make the whole memory of what just happened go away, but instead it made the picture of his mocking expressions even stronger in my mind.

The tears came hard and fast. Like those summer storms in the North East. You knew the rain was pouring faster than the drains could handle and that a flood was inevitable. I remember those rains from my childhood...

The force of all this rejection and loneliness was backing up on me. At first, releasing the tears felt like it was bringing harm instead of relief.

Orange Cones and Lessons in Forgiveness

I caught my eyes in the rearview mirror. They were swollen with sickness, overmedication and the deep ache of loneliness.

And that's when I stared into my own eyes and said the words that I didn't premeditate:

"This looks like a 'No' but it's a 'Not here. Not now', Stacey. This is a sign … There is a 'Yes' waiting somewhere for you. This is just not it. This is not where your 'Yes' is. This is an Orange Cone and it's *for* your good … "

That's when the whole idea of Orange Cones came to me.

If it weren't for the idea of Orange Cones, it would have been easy to hate Dr. Tom. Or the other dozen or so doctors who mis-diagnosed me, told me I was dying, or told me there was no hope for living fully, having children, or being well.

It was a long two years of misdiagnosis.

And a lot of resentment could have built up where healing was needed, if not for that picture of the Orange Cones.

See, Orange Cones are great for two reasons: they protect the people who are doing the work by creating a barrier around them. And secondly, the cones communicate to the drivers to "Go around!"

Orange cones don't do the work. They simply point to you, in their bright orange color to, "Go around."

Like that one doctor, who walked in to my room, took my symptoms and informed me that it sounded like a brain tumor and then walked right out of the exam room, leaving me completely alone and devastated. She was an Orange Cone.

Or the doctor, the Diplomat of Endocrinology, who told me, "I'm tired of messing with your thyroid medication, let's just take your thyroid out so that it won't be such a hassle for me." He was an Orange Cone.

Or the doctor who said, "Well, you're just making us all scratch our heads, Stacey. The only thing I can tell you is that what your body is doing, is what the body does right before it dies." Definitely an Orange Cone.

Every doctor who didn't have the answer was reminding me, "Go around me. I'm not the answer. Someone else is going to do the work."

Every "No" started becoming such a clear "Yes" to me, that everything in my life started looking like a "Yes."

"Yes, I'm the Orange Cone, go around."

"Yes, someone else is out there to help."

"Yes, I'm not the one for you today."

"Yes, you're moving in the right direction by figuring out I'm not your guy. Keep going."

Orange Cones and Lessons in Forgiveness

What a gift. To know that these people were not the answer and to go around them because an answer was waiting elsewhere.

I found the coolest, kick-back, non-alarmist doctor up at UCLA who actually took my TSH, T3, T4, Reverse T3 AND my TPO (Thyroid Peroxidase Antibodies).

And I did find the answer: an autoimmune dis-ease, called Hashimoto's.

He told me that I wasn't crazy.

And I found all these other really cool natural health professionals who have supported my life and fed into my well-being through nutrition and lifestyle changes.

And I found an avocation of almost 20 years – helping other folks in their health journeys, as that became one of my passionate missions in life.

The thing is this: instead of resentment and bitterness, I eventually had such gratitude. Wisdom was leading. I was learning to listen. What I was hearing was that every "No" was really my "Yes" waiting somewhere else.

And the gift of seeing the doctors (and other health professionals who didn't have the answer) as Orange Cones, allowed me to not only forgive them and love them, but it allowed me to truly appreciate them. They are doing a good work. They are helping other people in other ways and with other issues. Just not me, in mine.

You're Not Crazy and You're Not Alone

I'm so grateful to know where the answers are.
And where the answers are not.
Both are my gift.

Maybe it's time for you to take someone out of the category of
'The Asshole Who Didn't Help Me' and put them into the category of 'Orange Cone'.

You can even call them "Dr. Orange Cone" if you like. I mean, not
to their face. That wouldn't go over too well.

But just in your heart while you remember that every 'No' is a
'Yes' waiting somewhere else.

So, you just move along, little doggie, and bless that Dr. Orange
Cone while you walk out their door.

You can do it. Even in the middle of it being hard. In fact, that's
the most important place and time to do it. It sets you up to heal
faster, forgive more deeply, and to move on. You need that, more
than you need to attach a grudge to your heart and to your life.

So just bless every 'No' you get.

Because, every 'No' you walk away from
is just a 'Yes' you're walking toward.

Chapter 5

Supplements, The Saboteur, and The Messy Perfectionist

Supplements and I had a mutual understanding: I'd buy them, and then, I wouldn't take them.

Hashi's patients are famous for our vast list and counters full of supps – everything from A to Zinc – with essential oils, vitamins, flower essences, homeopathy, detoxifying clays, minerals and a few billion particles of probiotics thrown in, just for giggles.

It didn't matter if it was the crap vitamins I used to buy on the cheap that were more *fillers* than they were actual nutrients, or the highest grade that I would pay thousands of dollars in supplemental protocols – the consistent thing about me was that I didn't take them consistently.

It's been quite an interesting road of discovery of the reasons why I didn't take them. And guess what? I'm not alone. After talking to other Hashi's patients, I heard some of the same reasons for them, too.

You ready? Here we go...

You're Not Crazy and You're Not Alone

On Being a Perfectionist

One of the reasons I've not been consistent with my supps is the illusion of perfectionism.

I call the type of perfectionism I deal with as 'The Messy Perfectionist.'

I used to be the person to clean every corner, make everything perfect, all my t's crossed and my i's dotted. And then, my thyroid and adrenals took a Thelma and Louise kind of road trip and drove off the edge of a cliff.

I crashed.
I burned.
I was wiped out.

I was left with all that perfectionistic kind of standard, internally, but no ability to carry it out, externally.

I was too tired to clean the dishes, fix my hair, alphabetize the dust ...I just couldn't do it anymore.

My OCD was DOA.

I got sick. And I got fat.

Getting sick and fat really tattles on your belief system and your internal dialogue. Because, see...I didn't know that I had this perfectionistic/pass-or-fail kind of thinking until I couldn't keep up appearances in my body, my home, or my business life.

Supplements, The Saboteur, and The Messy Perfectionist

Everything was falling apart and getting ugly and I couldn't stop it. I couldn't keep up appearances. At all.

Sometimes I would wish that I had one of those hidden issues where I could still look pretty and have a clean house, but I didn't. This Hashimoto's thing not only kicked my butt physically, but because of that, it really forced me to look at what was inside of me, running my show.

I wanted to look good.
Always be on time.
Anticipate your needs.
Exceed your expectations.
And have a good reputation.

Those aren't bad things, but the reasons that I wanted them weren't healthy. I was afraid of failing, of disappointing you, of being seen as incompetent, of making you not like me for reasons that were within my control.

I was afraid of being rejected.

I held a harsh standard for myself
And assumed you did, too.

We do that, you know -- we project onto others what judgments we carry within. If we're being punitive about ourselves, we'll either think that others are being that way with us OR we will find people who actually ARE punitive with us.

It makes sense to me that this 'me, being hard on me' thinking shows up as an autoimmune disease – where our body sees itself as an enemy. How can they not be related? The fact that we spent years rejecting ourselves, defining ourselves by our weaknesses, and hating ourselves for our own imperfections – our own humanity.

How could autoimmune issues, where our body sees a part of us (our thyroid) that is actually a friend but calls it a 'foe', not be related to our self-hatred? How can it not be connected to the way we would punish ourselves for being so disappointing?

We push and push – and push ourselves some more -- well beyond our limits, without acknowledging the messages that our body sends us to slow down and to rest.

That is a form of self-rejection.

Whether this originated from a parent, teacher, coach, priest, rabbi or People Magazine, I don't know … Whether we entered from the other realm with this issue from some past life, or we chose to have this, I am unclear. All I can say is that I notice a pattern with Hashimoto's and other autoimmune patients, that they are chronically hard on themselves.

It reminds me of that meme I've seen floating around Facebook:

"AUTOIMMUNE DISEASE: because the only one strong enough to kick my ass is ME!"

Yeah.

Perfectionism sucks.

Supplements, The Saboteur, and The Messy Perfectionist

Unworthiness and Entitlement

And I'm going to go off on a tangent by saying this too: people who are usually very hard on themselves in certain areas, also indulge in great entitlement in other areas.

Let me explain that for a sec.

That insight came to me years ago: entitlement and unworthiness are two sides of the same coin – or two ends of the same spectrum, if you will.

Here's the backstory: one day, I was sitting in a green room with some of the other leaders of this music team I was hired to direct. We were deep in a brainstorming conversation and a head peeked in through the crack in the door. It was a woman, one of the singers on my team. She was a fair singer, but super committed to being there and giving her all.

Her eyes widened and she made a huge deal of sneaking in, knees high in the air in a comical way, stepping like The Pink Panther trying to avoid a land mine, "I'm so sorry! Oh my god! I had NO idea you were meeting! I NEVER would have come this way if I had known. I just have to get my coffee mug, so sorry! Actually, it's my husband's coffee mug, but it's from his work so, he really needs to bring it back..." We all just stared at her. "I'll be out of your hair in just a second. Don't mind me!"

She would *not* shut up.

Her insecurity and discomfort drew so much attention to her that all of us were completely distracted.

Yet, just a week before, she had been complaining that she never gets a solo and that's she's so balls-to-the-wall committed but was constantly getting passed up on one opportunity after another. She didn't have an accurate read on her ability to sing and thought she deserved more.

When she finally left the green room, the leadership team looked to me and asked, "Why does she do that? Get mad about not getting a vocal solo but then, act like such an inconvenience?"

I said something that hit me clearly in that moment, "Because unworthiness and entitlement are two ends of the same spectrum – and both come from fear. If she really knew how truly amazing she was, she wouldn't act that way. Love is balanced. It knows when to step forward and when to step back. Fear doesn't – so it swings from one extreme to another."

It was a profound moment for me to see my patterns lived out in her example. I was no different than her in my thinking, even though my actions were more easily hidden – at that time. For example, in my marriage: I didn't feel deserving of my husband's love and attention but, I wanted all of it.

I didn't want to take my supplements to get better because I felt unworthy of being well. And yet, I wanted to be able to eat anything I wanted without having a consequence.

It was in my life, too.

I know that was a tangent, but I seriously had to go there because it changed my life to see that Unworthiness and Entitlement were two sides of the same coin – and were something that I was going to need to address in my own life.

Back to messy perfectionism...

Perfectionism has a lot to do with a Fear of Rejection. And I was letting Fear of Rejection run my life.

When we're in Fear-mode, we live on adrenaline. We're amped up on the 'juice' we get from being in 'fight-or-flight' mode. It's energizing and electrifying. Until, you know, it drives off the edge of a cliff and leaves you with nothing and your adrenal glands get totally burned out.

So, before my adrenaline burnout, I was using my fight or flight juice to fuel my performance-driven, perfectionistic ways.

I stayed up late and would get up early to get all my work done. I'd make promises to please people who hung their acceptance of me on the thread of my performance. I'd burn out my health and, at times, my marriage just to keep those promises to people who couldn't have cared less about me.

But when my life crashed and burned, I couldn't hold my appearances together. All of those plates that I had been spinning, started shattering, one-by-one. And then, some a few at a time until I was standing there, 270 lbs., my skin a mess, my life a mess. My everything – a mess.

Ergo, The Messy Perfectionist

The Gifts in the Middle of the Mess

My gift of being a visual person who appreciates beauty, along with my weakness for being vain, both came together and forced me to look at my shit. Because honestly, if my life – and body – hadn't been falling apart in front of my eyes, I may have been tempted to keep going. I could have just kept living in an un-examined mess of issues that were dressed in pretty packages, because I was sadly content with things 'looking good.'

That's part of why I can't help but be grateful for this diagnosis. Because all the external things falling apart have been signposts for me to look at what's been breaking down on the inside.

And I do personally believe that I was breaking down on the in-side, long before the external consequences showed up.

What does this have to do with supplement taking?

If I missed even one pill, at one time, on one day, I felt I'd failed, ruined it, kaput. And then, I'd have to start over. Pass or Fail. Good girl/Bad Girl. If I didn't do it (whatever 'it' was) then, I had ruined everything.

(Not) taking supplements helped me see the perfectionist in me.

The Illusion of the Perfect Day

I had that same thing with diets years ago: if I planned on starting a diet on Monday (you know, the magical day to start a diet) and

Supplements, The Saboteur, and The Messy Perfectionist

I started Monday off with, I don't know – say a brownie … or five -- I'd have to wait 'til the next Monday to try again. In between, of course, I'd eat a weeks worth of 'Last Suppers' to prepare for the next diet attempt. Gain 6 pounds to lose 2 = bad math.

I've even done that on New Years Day – I'd take my New Year's Resolutions and then, break them within 12 minutes of the new year and say, "Okay, well, I'll try again next year."

Crazy, I know, but it made sense to the way my perfectionistic mind was working. At one point several years ago, I decided that wasn't working for me and I took on a new mindset. One that said, 'I know the holiday is coming in three weeks but I don't have to eat myself silly until that point. What if I stopped waiting for all the holidays to be over and I just ate really clean. And then, had that holiday be my day of indulgence?'

It was like a brand new thought. I had an epiphany, the angels sang and I started losing weight, being healthier, and having great holidays. I stopped trying to be perfect and waiting for the perfect day or the perfect eating plan and I started living in greater freedom.

Again – you're asking, what does that have to do with supplements?

Because maybe you feel like you've ruined it and you've got those almost full bottles (or, gasp! unopened bottles!) of pills on the counter and you're waiting for the next Monday to take them. Or you're waiting for the next doctor to tell you what to do. Or you're waiting for the next trend of supplements to come along before you start taking them. But my advice is to start now.

You're Not Crazy and You're Not Alone

Marla Cilley of FLYLady fame (www.flylady.net) is a great example to me. Marla started a cleaning protocol for overwhelmed, messy perfectionistic women by breaking the housework down into bite-sized bits and giving folks routines to follow for their housekeeping.

Her name FLYLady stands for Finally Loving Yourself.

One of the ways she encourages people to love themselves is by taking care of their home. She's all about letting go of the perfectionism she had formerly dealt with. Marla has two great sayings that I particularly love, "Even an imperfectly cleaned house is a blessing to my family." And "You're not behind, so don't try to catch up. Just jump in where you are."

So ... you didn't start the supplements yesterday and you missed a few today? No big whoop. You're not behind – you don't have to be perfect. Just jump in where you are. And keep going, it's going to make a difference.

On Being Overwhelmed

I hate horse pills. I don't love swallowing pills. And I'm not good at taking pills.

I'm a barrel of laughs, I tell you.

This is coming from someone, who as a child, used to swallow ice cubes, pretzels or saltine crackers in big chunks just to see how much she could swallow without having to chew.

Supplements, The Saboteur, and The Messy Perfectionist

At some point, I grew up and developed a fear of choking. (I've also heard that I'm not alone in that as a Hashi's person.)

It would be so daunting for me. I'd go to see a specialist, spend $500 for the visit and another $700 on a supplement protocol (all not covered by insurance, thank you very much) and I'd come home and stare at the bottles on my counter while I tried to not have an anxiety attack.

Then, with my brain working the way it was, I couldn't figure out which ones were before breakfast, how long I had to wait before taking my thyroid pill, which ones I had to take with food, which ones weren't supposed to be taken after 4 p.m. and which ones were supposed to be taken on the third full moon of the solstice.

I mean really. Take a stressed person, with a foggy brain, give them a scrillion bottles with tiny labels and lots of instructions and it's pretty much a recipe for disaster.

My husband would stand there and watch me, watching the bottles. He'd gently touch my back so as to not startle me, "You know... they don't open themselves and jump into your mouth." Or his other famous line, "You know, they don't work in your body when they're sitting on the counter. You have to actually *take* them to make them work."

I know. The truth was, I was just overwhelmed.

That's why I LOVED when I went to see Dr. Koren Barrett, one of my naturopaths, for the very first time. She looked at my labs, listened to my symptoms and said, "Well, we are not going to detox you at all. Not yet. You're a mom of two young boys and you need to feel good. You haven't felt that way for a long time."

She leaned forward over her clipboard, "We need to get you feeling good again."

Oh my god, I wanted to kiss this woman full on the lips for understanding.

Then, she started writing the supplements I had to take and I wanted to take back that kiss.

I started to sweat.
The room got hazy.
And I felt a little woozy.

But then, she stopped.

I looked down. The list was short.

"That's all?" I asked.

It was manageable. I could do this.

She nodded, "Let's start with these and we'll take it from there."

     - Pantothenic Acid
     - 5 HTP
     - Selenium
     - B Complex
     - Vitamin D

That was it. I felt so understood. I had been in a brain fog for months. I had been dizzy for almost a year and depressed for I couldn't remember how long.

I took my supplements faithfully (notice I said 'faithfully' and not 'perfectly' meaning I did forget some on some days, but I jumped back in when I forgot.)

Within three weeks, I started feeling significantly better.

With enough hope and a clear head under my belt two months later, I started making food changes. With the clarity and wellness I started experiencing from that, I started refining my food choices and adding other supplements or switching old ones out for new ones. Within about a year I did a detox and ended up feeling great (after a few wonky days, which were to be expected) and now have, what I would call a "healthy lifestyle."

Sitting in our states of overwhelm and perfectionism get us nowhere fast. Taking baby steps in a direction, with some kind of regularity can affect changes that lead us to greater and greater transformations.

FLYLady had a breakdown after a death in her family and a divorce from her husband. She went to a 10-day treatment program, and the first assignment the other ladies had was to give her a makeover. They took her depressed state, stringy, oily hair and frumpy clothing and perked her up with a new look.

When she left there, she felt well enough to put together a morning routine of three items to do, and afternoon routine of three items to do and an evening routine of three items to do – all to keep her house and life in order.

You're Not Crazy and You're Not Alone

It took her 9 months because she took one baby step at a time to implement those changes. These have ended up serving her, and now millions of other women, for life.

I'm not telling you to take the supplements that I took. What works for me, may not work for you. And plus, certain supps make better sense in certain seasons so, me telling you what to take is not what this section is about. I'm not even telling you to take any, because maybe you want really great foods to be your 'supplements.' Awesome.

(Logistically though, one thing I do believe is that if you do take supps, you should research really clean, organic products when-ever possible, with the least amount of fillers that you can. It's wise to check and make sure that your supplements are free of any allergens you have sensitivity to. Wheat and soy get hidden into stuff – Hashimoto's buyer, beware.)

Ultimately, when you're dealing with being overwhelmed, it's about working with someone who knows you, understands you and is going to help you take baby steps.

Once you get into a place of feeling well enough, you'll be able to do other things that bring you toward greater health. Finding someone who helped me out of the state of overwhelm, like Dr. Barrett, and into baby stepping my way into the next level of health, was a gift in my life.

On Being a Self-Saboteur

If I don't talk about this, I feel like this monster could keep lurking in the shadows and we'd be missing a huge part of the equation.

For people who are used to dealing with one stormy season of life after another, combined with a belief system that says you're not worth anything good happening, taking supplements can be a trigger for that unworthiness monster to be unleashed.

Let me give you an example in another direction: you step on the scale and you lose another 4 lbs. and are closer to your goal weight than you've ever been. And suddenly, you want to eat your weight in classic potato chips and chocolate-glazed donut holes.

It's not that you really are craving them. It's that the part of you that doesn't know how to live in the good parts of life, and feels more comfortable going through hard times, is kicking into high gear.

There's a part of your belief system that includes sabotaging you.

Same with supplements. As soon as a practitioner says, "Here, take this Vitamin D3, it helps with depression, weight loss, blood sugar issues, sleep ..." Which are *exactly your* issues, you find yourself avoiding the Vitamin D, losing the bottle and leaving it in your rental car that you returned before flying home to Michigan.

Yeah. That's no mistake. That's the self-sabotage monster.

It's the part of me that is pretty sure I'm not worth being well, and is pretty convinced that good stuff isn't for me, and that feels pretty confident that the minute I start enjoying some of the good life then, something bad is going to happen and it's all going to be taken away.

It's the whole fuck-me, Charlie Brown and Lucy scenario where she holds the ball and promises she'll let him kick it this time. So good ol' CB finally screws up enough courage, hope and trust (all which had been crushed several times before) to run toward it and she pulls it away… again.

So, since life's going to end up shitty anyway, why not just skip the middle man of 'happiness' and 'hope' and let's just keep things miserable, instead. At least that's familiar and I know my way through that.

Right?

So sad.

I know that I've not been alone in those beliefs.
I know that many of you have been there, too.

When I take my supplements, for me, it's not just about putting something good in my system. It's also about pushing past the story of my unworthiness and taking actions that are different than the feelings that have been lying to me. It's me saying to that old tape that runs in my head, 'I'm not letting you run my show anymore.'

It's me loving myself.

I believe we were born to love ourselves, but someone or something in our life retrained us to live in fear and unworthiness instead.

Supplements, The Saboteur, and The Messy Perfectionist

Someone lied to us.
And we believed it.
We don't have to keep perpetuating the lie.

The Self-Saboteur and Hope

And for many of us, we learned to live without hope.

To eat healing foods, to drink healing water and to take healing supplements is addressing something else that is huge for us: it's addressing the fact that we didn't believe we had a future to even be here for.

Many of us planned an escape route of an early death in our minds. I'm not talking about suicide, specifically, though that has been a very real thought for many with thyroid issues. Which shouldn't be surprising: I remember my friend, who had been an FBI agent and had a great passion for natural health, she had this inclination to ask for autopsies on suicide victims and to have a report made about the state of their thyroid. She was told on every. single. autopsy. that the suicide victim had either an atrophied thyroid the size of a pea or it was completely non-existent.

Yes, depression, doom, and hopelessness are directly affected by our thyroids. And I believe it also may have been part of the fabric of our beliefs before we had thyroid issues. I'm not sure how that lands for you, but here's the thing you should know about me and this book: you don't have to agree with everything in it to get something valuable out of it.

That was a little tangent, sorry. Valuable and a tangent.

You're Not Crazy and You're Not Alone

Back to the horrible subject of suicide: I'm not talking about taking ourselves out of the picture via suicide. I'm talking about writing ourselves out of our future – not believing we'll be there to see our silver or golden anniversary, not believing we'll hold our grandbabies, not believing the good life and a future is for us.

That hopelessness is profound that we have dealt with, and that sense of doom, is something many have dealt with for years.

For me, when I had gone through a terrible sexual abuse by two different people when I was 12 – 14 years old, I found myself obsessed with death. I couldn't picture myself alive to see 16. And then, 18. And then, 21. And then 25.

Finally, I was at dinner with a good friend who happens to be a marriage/family counselor and knew my story and I asked him why he thought that was. He said, "Stacey, you were writing an end to something that felt endless. We do that when the pain of what we're going through seems like it's never going to stop and life is out of our control. We choose an end to the suffering by imagining our death. As a young girl, you didn't know when the abuse would stop so, you wrote your own ending."

I thought there was something brilliant about what he said, and it resounded in me.

So, all these years, I still haven't had a picture of me being 30, or having my first child or my 20th anniversary. I'm 44 now, have two children and am entering my 25th year of marriage.

I've determined that having a picture of my future isn't necessary to me having a future. I've (mostly) stopped being superstitious about it and tell myself instead, "I'm evolving so quickly that any picture of myself in my head would be out of date by tomorrow!" I'm playing a little and it sounds silly but, if we're going to make up a story about our future, it might as well be an empowering one, right?

Supplements and the Spiritual Practice

For me, taking supplements is a spiritual practice that is rerouting me back to my original design of loving and being loved. It's that spiritual Vitamin Self-Love that is a true healer in this whole game.

Loving myself means actually participating in my possible wellness and health.

You know what emotionally and mentally healthy people do? When they hear from a trusted source that something is good for them, they look into it and they do it.

When someone who doesn't love herself hears that something's good for her, she assumes it's for the other people who are more worthy and she runs in a corner and hides.

Or eats herself into a catatonic state.

Or keeps herself so busy she has no time to take care of herself.

Or she buys supplements and stares at them sitting on her counter.

You're Not Crazy and You're Not Alone

Yeah. That.

I am learning to love myself: one day, one meal, one relationship, one meditation, one nap and even one supplement at a time.

Now, put this fabulous book down, pour yourself a glass of water and take a supplement or two.

Come on now.

Don't just stare at me or the counter full of supplements. They're not going to open themselves and jump in your mouth.

And neither am I.

Which just sounds ridiculous enough that I'm keeping that sentence in there.

So come on now, go partner in your healing, your wellness and your future.

And please, don't make me send my husband over there.

He's got his hands full with

Little Miss

*'You
Know
Who.'*

Chapter 6

Sleep, Rest, and Other Mysteries of Life

I could have easily called this chapter, "How come I'm too tired to do anything, but not tired enough to go to sleep?"

Heck, I could have made that the title for the entire book.

Seriously, if I had a nickel for every time someone posted on a Hashi's page, "Does anybody else deal with insomnia?" I'd be writing this chapter from my own private island off the Gulf of Somewhere Fabulous.

Yes.

Exhaustion AND insomnia can be two of the bedfellows (pardon the completely insensitive pun) to Hashimoto's.

Having my thyroid go wonky-doo and eating the wrong foods led me to experience exhaustion like I had never known before. My eyeballs were scratchy, my body ached all over, and I felt like someone had strapped 50 lb. weights to each of my legs.

I'd say to my husband, "I feel like a really fat Barbie Doll with sag-gy boobs and no Barbie Dream House to find some comfort in. It's like somebody took off my legs and put them on backwards."

You're Not Crazy and You're Not Alone

(I used to do that to my Barbie, just for kicks. I'd take her legs out of the hip joints and put them on the other way so that her butt was facing front and her legs and feet were pointed back.

Not sure why I did that when I was a kid, but apparently there's Barbie-karma and let me tell you, it's a bitch.)

I felt terrible whether I slept for 10 hours or no hours -- like I was hit by a truck.

We all know how much sleep matters.

If you don't, sleep if affects your moods, your immune system, your blood pressure, your cortisol level, your weight, your desire for sex and so much more. Sleep is super important.

My girlfriend, Cathy, who was pregnant, called me years before my worst insomnia kicked in. She was not having an easy time of her pregnancy, "Stacey. I can't sleep. I'm ready to lose my mind!" The Wisdom that came to me was for her to embrace it, not resist it, and to trust that she'd have every bit of energy she needed for what she truly needed to get done.

Easy to say.

Here's what I've experienced about giving advice to friends who ask or when I'm counseling my clients: eventually, I have to live what I talk about for it to be taken out of the 'Theory' category and into the 'Fact' category. Experiencing my own advice also allows me to deliver it with the greatest amount of compassion and credibility.

I mean, really, that makes sense, right? I mean, who are you going to pick to lead you down the way of weight loss? A naturally skinny person who has no clue what it's like to find comfort, over a three-day weekend, in an entire Confetti Cake with blue frosting...

OR someone who has been heavy and depressed and then, found a way to lose the weight and is happy again?

Well, I had a sneaky feeling that the advice I had given to my friend on the subject of *sleep*, was the advice I was going to have to heed...

What Was I Thinking?

A couple of years after my conversation with Cathy, we moved from the West Coast to the East Coast. We were going for a two-year commitment to this little church, in this little village in Upstate New York. My boys were young and the opportunity really appealed to our sense of adventure so, despite it being an intrinsically busy time, we decided to add the chaos of a cross-country move to our lives.

On the practical, job-end of things, we were there to do music and speaking, but we quickly discovered that we were there for so much more.

Soon after we arrived, I started getting sick.

It began with one UTI after another followed by antibiotics (which I hadn't been on in years since Dr. Orange Cone had overdone it with me) with one challenging reaction after another. That led to my gut being a mess again and a whole host of other new symptoms that I was dealing with: fevers, trembling, hair falling out, skin rashes ... it was a whole lot of 'not fun.'

Now, this was seven years past my hypothyroid diagnosis, five years past my Hashimoto's diagnosis. Despite all I had read, tried, and learned there was still so much more I had yet to experience and discover with this whole autoimmune thing.

I still didn't understand the fuller breadth of Hashimoto's. The revelations about food sensitivities and gluten-free hadn't come to me just yet. I was still in the mode of 'you take your thyroid pill, your probiotics, and your aged garlic and you *should* be feeling better.'

And I was also in the mode of, 'Well, of course you're tired – you just moved across North America and have two little squirts who are nursing and almost never sit still.'

Duh.

So, I just thought 'sick and tired' were normal and par for the course.

In the midst of all the exhaustion and sickness, I started questioning if this had been the best time for me to take on a new stressful commitment with two moves, back and forth across the country, in two years' time. Probably not.

But then again, knowing life and how it works out, it was probably the perfect time.

Sleep, Rest, and Other Mysteries of Life

Sleepless in New York

Now, it was my turn to not sleep. I hadn't slept than more 3 or 4 broken hours a night since I had been pregnant with my second son – just like Cathy when she was pregnant with her second son. I had a saying that, I'm pretty sure, could go down in history: *broken sleep is like no sleep.*

I'd walk through the day like a zombie, feeling like a complete failure for being too tired to be kind, to do the laundry, to clean the house, and to make the meals in a consistent June Cleaver fashion.

I also think that when my second son came out the chute, my desire for sex must have snuck out of my body and escaped down the fire exit.

So, yeah. There wasn't a whole lot of good vibration in that area, either.

Yeah. I just wrote that.

And I'm leaving it.

It was all kinds of fun in my body.

So, after a full day of feeling like a failure, I'd go to bed and stare at the ceiling.

Awake.

Able to replay, in full color, how I had been such a loser all day.

You're Not Crazy and You're Not Alone

(Even though I wasn't, you know? It's just that whole 'thinking you're an awful person if you're not a perfect person' bullshit lie that so many of us women deal with.)

To be so very, very tired and to not be able to sleep was its own stress. Then, to add to it, feeling like failure of a woman. And *then*, just to top it off, the pressure of being a working, nursing mom was overwhelming.

I've never been so good at math as when I was figuring out how many hours of sleep I *wasn't* going to be getting before the kids woke up.

"Hi Stacey, I'd Like to Introduce You to Your Adrenal Glands."

It was one thing to have this thyroid thing in my late twenties, *before* having kids. It was a whole different game, having two young, busy boys while I was in my mid-thirties.

My dear friend, Nancy from Alaska, who was a spiritual counselor and had also been a nurse in her career, was listening to my symptoms in our weekly counseling calls.

She came across a book and suggested that I look into it: "Adrenal Fatigue: The 21st Century Stress Syndrome" by James Wilson and Jonathan V. Wright.

I had not really heard of Adrenal Fatigue but when I got that hot, little book in my hands, it became my Bible. The symptoms I had were in there: body trembling, skin burning, random fevers, exhaustion, brain fog, chronic infections, emotional overload and more. The struggles I had were right in there. And the sleeplessness and zero desire for sex … yup. Those were in there, too!

According to Dr. Wilson: "Adrenal fatigue (hypoadrenia) is a collection of signs and symptoms, known as a syndrome, that results when the adrenal glands function below the necessary level. Most commonly associated with intense or prolonged stress, it can also arise during or after acute or chronic infections, especially respiratory infections such as influenza, bronchitis or pneumonia. As the name suggests, its paramount symptom is fatigue that is not relieved by sleep.

When your adrenal glands function, but not well enough to maintain optimal homeostasis because their output of regulatory hormones has been diminished - usually by over-stimulation. Over-stimulation of your adrenals can be caused either by a very intense single stress, or by chronic or repeated stresses that have a cumulative effect." (www.adrenalfatigue.org)

And I also learned, from experience, that your adrenal glands can feel like they're a different time zone than you are. When the kids come home from school and you need energy at 3:30 p.m., you have none. When you're ready to go to bed at 11 p.m., you can't shut your eyes.

Yeah, I was Living the Dream.

Apparently, the stress of so many physical changes, plus the demands of family, and the move threw my body into a tailspin. And that was probably on top of all the other stressors in my life since I was a child.

Someone described adrenal fatigue as living in 'fight or flight' mode, adrenaline surging, as if you were being chased by a bear. All the time.

My life pretty much felt like a bear was chasing me. From an adrenal standpoint, I lived, running for my life.

The Relationship/Performance Factor

It also seemed to coincide with a breakdown in some of my relationships: I was having a tough time with two key family members and our new boss at the church.

Plus, Rock and I were in that awkward, exhausted transition of being new parents to two little guys in less than two years time. We hadn't found our rhythm yet and that perfect storm of being tired grown-ups, with little sleep and less sex made for more tension.

Oh, and my relationship with God... did I mention that teeny-tiny detail that he and I were in a breakdown, too?

See, at some point in New York, I stopped being able to perform – for my family of origin, for my little growing family, for the new church where I was working, and for God.

I couldn't help but notice that so many areas of my life were crashing and burning: my physical, my spiritual, my emotional, and my relational life.

I had been through hard times before that were a lot, but it just stood out differently in New York. The reason it was all so glaringly obvious is because the little village where we had moved to, was quiet. And since we were new and weren't well-known there, we didn't have our demanding social life like in Southern California. We weren't running from one fabulous event after another. The phone wasn't ringing off the hook – or almost at all. The Internet connection barely ever worked. It was like we were in social quarantine.

We weren't distracted.

I mean, life was crazy in its own way, don't get me wrong. But it was quiet enough on the outside, that I got start hearing all that noise going on inside my head.

In that space of so much silence, I started seeing how messed up things were inside of me. I started questioning a lot of things about my life: my spirituality and the specific theologies behind my beliefs, as well as the general questions of what was motivating me to do the things that I was doing.

Here I had moved 3,000 miles to work at our new job, where I was supposed to care for and serve people. All I really wanted to do was run for the hills and live naked in a cave until I sorted out what was stirring inside of me. (Naked, for no other reason than the fact that I didn't want to do any. more. laundry.)

In a weird way, the insomnia helped. I mean, the downside of insomnia is that you're incredibly and overwhelmingly exhausted, leading to high anxiety. The upside is that while everyone else is sleeping, you have a whole lot of time to hang out with your thoughts and to see how crazy they are.

You're Not Crazy and You're Not Alone

In the back of my mind were my words to Cathy, beckoning me:

Embrace.
Don't Resist.
Trust.

That was easy for me to say except I had two kids who looked to me as their food source and camp director. A husband who planned on me being an active partner in this whole 'Life' thing. And a new job that was waiting for me to be a light in their dark places through my music.

And, oh yeah ... a dining room with seven layers of ugly wallpaper for me to scrape off.

I was sick.
My family still needed me.
My job needed me.

But I was unraveling.

Not sleeping, night after night, became a platform for one anxiety attack after another, with brief episodes of intense introspection.

It was lovely.
So relaxing.
Not.

In the middle of it all, I believe I was being called to 'rest.'

Sleep, Rest, and Other Mysteries of Life

The Call to Rest

The call to *rest* showed up in a few unbelievably miraculous ways which I wrote about in another book, God Loves Me, I Think…Stories from Hell, Heaven, and the Other Side of Texas so, I won't go into all of that here but I do want to share about this one significant moment.

It showed up one day when we had just moved into that old brick house in New York. A neighbor came over and said kindly and matter-of-factly, "Just wanted you to know, you have to boil the water." I scrunched my nose and was like, *Huh? I moved to another place in America, not to a Third World country …*

He nodded, "The water gets turbid on account of the rain and the poor fittings on the pipes underground so, just be sure to boil the water. Oh and you may need to skim it too. Well, welcome to the neighborhood and have a good night!"

I closed the door and stood in my dining room full of boxes and no furniture and looked up to the ceiling where God lives, "You're kidding right? I move all this way with two kids and a husband who, thankfully hasn't cut me up into tiny pieces and left me on the side of the road for getting us into this mess, and now, we have to boil the water? I don't think so. I didn't sign up for Little House on the Prairie, thank you very much."

I walked to the kitchen, threw a pot for spaghetti in the sink and turned on the spigot and let it run for a good half a minute.

It looked great. Clean as a whistle. I turned the water off. *Our neighbor must be nuts…*

I went to the other side of the kitchen to futz with the stove. After a few tries, I got the old gas stove lit and went to get the pot of water from the sink. The water had settled and there it was: This mess of brown, foamy, gross water just staring at me.

And that's when it hit me,

"Shit.
That's *me*."

I look fine when I'm running and going a million miles an hour but then, I settle down and you can see what's really there.

My internal waters were dark and turbid.

I pulled up the only chair in the kitchen and sat down,

I leaned forward, "Okay God, what do we do? Should I read more, pray more, help more? You just tell me and I'll do it." I was used to pulling up my sleeves and putting more elbow grease into life when something didn't work.

I'm not entirely sure how to describe what it sounds like when The Creator of the Universe shakes his head, but I think I heard it that day, "No, Stacey. You just rest, I'll do the work."

Trusting, When You Don't Trust, So You Can Learn To Trust – Huh?

It was uncomfortable to think about sitting back, after I had spent so many years keeping myself busy with good and noble pursuits to cover up the fact that I felt terrible about myself.

Which, by the way, no one calls you on when you're doing noble stuff. Very few people go, "Oh Stacey, you're just helping too much, you need to take time off." No, it's just the opposite, "Oh you're so responsible, now can you do MORE?"

And it's not like I had a side-job of being a bank robber or prostitute where someone would say, "Hmmm … that seems a tad self-destructive. How about we chat about what you're running away from … "

Nope. I was a good person. Doing good things.

I couldn't see that even all my participation in noble activities was part of my cover-up.

Until I rested.

But "Rest" was quickly becoming my four-letter word. And here's why:

I didn't know how to rest because, ultimately, what I learned is that rest is about trust.

And I didn't trust.

When you are able to truly rest, whether it's going through your own health stuff, or watching your spouse grow through their crap, or your kids go through puberty and they have friends who seem weird, or you're tired and you want to lay your head down for a good night's sleep …

You're Not Crazy and You're Not Alone

Trust is what you need in order to do all of that.

Surrender.
Letting go of control.
Any of that sound familiar?

Anyone out there have a control issue or three?
Or is it just me...

Sigh.

So many of us with Hashimoto's have trust issues: it may have started with that family of origin stuff, where you couldn't trust you were safe in your own home -- but then, it turned into grown-up stuff:

- Not being able to trust your spouse was committed to you.
- Not being able to trust that your doctor was giving you the correct information, or the whole scoop on what you were dealing with.
- Not being able to trust that your family wouldn't turn on you in your time of need.
- Not being able to trust that God was there for you and wanted good things for you.
- Not being able to trust that if you didn't do it, it would still get done.
- Not being able to trust life's process.
- Not being able to trust yourself.

One of the most common themes I have heard over years of counseling women is: 'I don't trust that if I actually sit down and let myself relax, that I'll ever get up again.'

Sleep, Rest, and Other Mysteries of Life

Women were afraid to slow down, because if they did, they'd fall down and completely fall apart. And all that would be left were the remnants of a broken woman who used to be a contribution to life, but now she wasn't.

It's a terrible fear to have, especially when you've tied your worth to your work.

I understand that.
So well.

I was the most restless person being called to 'rest.'

Fear and Restlessness

Fear and inner restlessness go together.

There was so much fear driving my train.

Fear doesn't trust.
Fear tries to control.

What happens to many of us with Hashimoto's and Adrenal Fatigue/Exhaustion?

We lose control. The very thing we fear (surrendering) comes upon us in the form of losing control, because we simply can't manage and maintain everything we used to. All those plates that we were spinning start crashing to the ground in rather unceremonious, uncomfortable ways.

We're forced to lay everything down, simply because we can't hold it all any more.

In the middle of all this big motion of moving to New York and learning how to put little people in snowsuits (that was fun. Not.), I was now being called to *rest*. I just couldn't do my life that same way anymore, not spiritually and not physically.

I was fried.

The Practice of Resting

So, I started a practice of resting 15 minutes a day. I'd sit on our back porch in New York and look at the Northern Spruce trees. I'd try to pray, sing or read something from my religious background. If it sounds like I was still trying to 'do' more than I was simply 'being', you're right. I was still trying to perform. Even in the middle of resting.

I'd sit, shifting in my seat once every twelve seconds, wanting to lose my mind. I was like that kid in class who won't sit still. And even though my lips weren't moving, my thoughts were going non-stop:

Is this okay?
Am I doing this right?
How will I know when we're done?'
Are we done yet?

I'd just kind of hear the Divine say, in the most holy and kind way, "Just shut up, Stacey. Just shhhhh..."

Sleep, Rest, and Other Mysteries of Life

When the weather got too cold to sit outside, I'd set the timer and point to my husband as I walked to our bedroom, "I'm going to go rest. If I come out before the timer goes off, shoot me." His eyes would get wide, "Don't you think that's a little much?" I'd shake my head because I was taking this seriously. Then, I'd lock my door and lie on my bed tapping my fingers, thinking about all the dishes in the sink that I could be washing, and all the clothes I could be folding...

My mind would spin unmercifully. There was so much noise inside my head.

Thoughts about how bad I was, or how mad I was – and how guilty I felt for being bad and mad – and what a disappointment I was to God and my family. It was a constant barrage, replaying conversation after conversation where I had felt like I had blown it with someone and the 20 ways I should have said or done *it* better. I could see nothing good in me.

No wonder I didn't want to slow down. Look what happened when I did ...

All of this turmoil and rejection was inside of me but I couldn't see it for what it was during all those years when I kept myself so busy. Because I kept moving my body with over-activity and over-commitment. I kept my mind distracted and couldn't hear this inner noise.

The beeping would go off after 15 minutes and I felt like I was being let out of prison.

I didn't know how to be alone with myself.

I didn't know how to *rest.*

Because I didn't know how to *trust.*

I didn't really see how restless I was internally, until I took on the practice of resting externally.

I was in the habit of using my workaholic ways to mask the truth that I was really afraid of life.

I was afraid of love.

I was afraid of God.

It was a good thing I was being called to *rest* around the time my adrenals were driving off the edge of a cliff. My spirit needed a break and so did my body. The process was wildly uncomfortable but the timing was perfect.

The Physical Component

Dr. Wilson's book on Adrenal Fatigue was a perfect companion during those two years (and beyond) because hormones and adrenal fatigue are super important to look into as a reason you're not sleeping.

Those lifestyle changes that he noted in his book were brilliant aids for me. I started getting rid of complicated, toxic relationships. I started the habit of getting to bed by 10 p.m. whether I was asleep or not. I started drinking my salted water in the morning (to help support the adrenal glands) and began doing things that made me happy during the day.

My religion hadn't valued happiness, it valued suffering and service *way* before happiness. Happiness was even seen as a "selfish" pursuit.

But I already didn't know how to take care of my own happiness, well before the religious component showed up in my life. I already had a habit of doing good things out of obligation. I had years of not being true to my heart. I had decades of not being good to me.

I had to start the conversation all over again of what really made me happy and what truly, was healthy.

I love Dr. Wilson's book because it was an integral part of my 'heath and happiness' conversation I needed to be in. I HIGHLY recommend it. The wisdoms are timeless even though it's almost 15 years old.

If you're wondering how much those two things go together – the spiritual burnout with the adrenal burnout, I did too. I wondered what would happen if we'd enter into a state of surrender and trust, how much that would aid our body in getting out of the 'Fight/Flight' mode and into a state where our bodies could heal.

My guess, and experience was that they're pretty connected.

Spiritual Rest

After a few months of resting almost daily, my mind was quieted. The noise had finally faded of that constant tape of 'What a bad person I am' and I learned how to be in the space of the silence.

In the new silence of my mind, I entered a thoughtful conversation with God and I asked a question in my resting time, "Would you show me who you are?"

I didn't get an answer on that. Not at first anyway.

Instead, thoughts and memories came to mind carrying insights. The first one was about arrogance: about how I had used arrogance to cover up my insecurity. After a month or so of meditating on the missing security in my life and a journey into some healing, the second revelation came:

Information on how I used judgment to help me feel more in control of a life that felt unwieldy. How labeling others was my way of putting handlebars onto a life that felt out of control and scary.

And after a month or two of coming to some inner healing about that, I got a third download about my pride. It wasn't the kind of pride that stood on the top of a hill and said, "Look how wonderful I am!" or "I'm better than everyone else!" No. It was the kind of pride that didn't trust that life was good and 'for' me. As a result, I lived thinking I had to do everything myself.

Arrogance.
Judgment.
Pride.

Sleep, Rest, and Other Mysteries of Life

All symptoms of my mistrust.

All the information came in the gentlest of ways. Without one hint of criticism or mean-spiritedness. Each revelation I heard made me want to say, "Thank you. Yes. That's true."

Hearing that truth and seeing it in the space of non-judgment about myself, freed me.

I learned how to be *with* me in those resting times. I couldn't wait to have them and I made them longer than 15 minutes – calling them my 'Rendezvous with God' time.

Eventually, my whole day and even into the night, I had this sense of abiding and loving companionship.

I realized that I had been living in my own perception of God based on the arrogance, judgment and pride I had. Those were the building blocks I had used to create (or embrace other people's ideas of) a punishing God.

I think of it like a windshield, actually – like you're driving with all this mud, dirt and grime on the window but mistakenly thinking all of this stuff *is* the view. Then, you realize, "Oh, THAT's not the view, that's the dirt keeping me FROM the view."

My idea of God was a figment of my perception. It was defined by the dirt on my window – the misbeliefs about god that were obstructing my vision. The dirt wasn't the vista I was longing to see. It was blocking me from seeing God clearly.

A new peace came to me. And while I didn't know who this God was, I knew he wasn't the asshole god I had believed in for such a long time.

Then, one night, in my state of peaceful insomnia, I heard Words with No Voice say, "I am Love." I nodded. It made so much sense because I had experienced such love from this conversation over those two years.

The Divine went on, "And you…are Love."

Tears came to me. Because it made so much sense. How could a God of Love make me and I not be Love myself? How could I be made from the fabric of the Beauty, Wisdom, and Wonder of the Divine and not have Beauty, Wisdom, and Wonder woven into the fabric of me?

It was so beautiful and I felt an alignment. My thinking lined up with a truth that made sense to me.

And satisfied me.

That night, I fell asleep. My husband woke me up eight hours later. He had a concerned on his face because, well … he thought I was dead since I hadn't slept that long in years.

I was both happy and sad: happy that I had reached a point of surrender spiritually and some restoration for my adrenals physically, but sad that I started sleeping through my rendezvous times.

This deep peace meant a deep trust. I believe both were a significant part that gave me deep sleep.

Sleep, Rest, and Other Mysteries of Life

I am Love.
And you are Love.

That journey is valuable: to look at what beliefs are running your life. To examine, in gentle ways, if there's a trust-less-ness behind your restlessness.

And to consider exploring a journey with the Divine in you so that you can live in a deeper trust and therefore, a deeper rest.

I want us all to experience the result: a sacred, deep, and abiding peace.

My Current Sleep and Rest

To this day, I still go through funny sleep patterns. Sometimes, I'll fall asleep at 7 p.m. and wake up at midnight, write for a few hours and then, sleep until morning. I love it!

And sometimes, I'll go to bed at 10 and sleep 'til 3. I'll lie there and meditate or do my Jin Shin Jyutsu practice of holding my fingers, which represent different emotions and different organs. It's super restful.

Sometimes, I'll go to bed at 9 and sleep straight through until 4, 5 or 6. I'll watch the trees out the window, put my hand on my husband's head as he sleeps and just feel gratitude for him.

Or sometimes, I'll pick up my phone and get all into checking Facebook and my e-mail. Welcome to my humanity!

You're Not Crazy and You're Not Alone

When my FB friends see my postings or hear about my sleep patterns, they think I'm nuts. They'll say things like, "God, Stacey! Don't you *ever* sleep?"

I give a couple of answers usually, one of them being about the whole idea of sleeping in shifts. It's even mentioned in the famous book, Canterbury Tales.

Back then, people slept for a few hours, woke an hour or two for prayer, meditation, sex, conversation with their spouse, and then, they'd return to the second shift of their sleep.

(http://slumberwise.com/science/your-ancestors-didnt-sleep-like-you)

That's one answer that I give to my FB friends who think I never sleep. But the best answer I can give to them is this:

I'm at peace with being awake, and I'm at peace with being asleep. I embrace the awake time. I don't resist it. And I trust that all the energy I need for the next day will be there when I need it.

Just like I told Cathy all those years ago, and lived out the learning myself, a few years later. Those words weren't a thin concept anymore, they were now thick yarn, woven into the tapestry of my *resting* experience.

So, yes, look into the Adrenal Fatigue book, and yes consider entering the deeper conversation of your restlessness, too. Your sleep and your rest, emotionally, physically, and spiritually matters.

Sleep, Rest, and Other Mysteries of Life

I'm not saying it's easy.
I'm saying it's worth it.

Let me restate that:

I'm not saying it's easy,
I'm saying
you're worth it.

Chapter 7

Liquids Make the World Go Round

I don't know what magic or science is going on, but sometimes, I drink a glass of water and I'm thirstier than when I started.

Has anyone had that happen or am I the cheese standing alone on this one?

You're at a party and there's a cooler full of wine, another full of beer, and still another full of water. I wave lovingly and longingly to the first two, and grab for the bottled water. I open it, take a big *glug* and my mouth instantly feels like I drank cotton.

Seriously, what's *that* about?

I have recognized that it's certain brands of water that make me feel that way.

I've also learned that it really matters what kind of liquids we drink, and that we drink a sufficient amount.

Dr. Batmanghelidj, author of The Body's Many Cries for Water describes how pains and symptoms in the body can actually be signs of not enough water when we're in a state of UCD (Unintentional Chronic Dehydration).

He states that simply by consuming enough pure water, we can help take care of issues like back pain, arthritis, heartburn and even unexpected areas like angina, high blood pressure, and high cholesterol.

(Check out: http://www.watercure.com/wondersofwater.html)

Liquids are essential when you have Hashimoto's. And I don't know about you, but there are two things I've noticed with having Hashimoto's:

1. I don't always feel like drinking something. I go through seasons where I struggle to get even 30 ounces in a day. I wonder if it's the depression part or the self-saboteur part. But honestly, I go through times where the last thing I want to have up to my lips is a bottle of water.

I have a theory, based on something I heard from some friends who live in Alaska. They do all these great, outdoor adventure sports when it's like a scrillion degrees below freezing.

(Have I ever mentioned that I'm allergic to winter? I do NOT. Like. Being. Cold.

Then again, I do NOT. Like. Being. Hot. *This* is why I live in Southern California.

But I digress...)

My Alaskan friends said that in the winter, thirst changes – making us *not* crave water, and therefore making it easier to dehydrate when we're cold. They make a concerted effort during their really, screamingly-long winter, to be sure to hydrate well.

I've wondered if, because our thyroid function is low and our body temperature is usually lower than the average bear, if that affects our desire to drink. Hmm…

2. I've noticed that I get underhydrated more easily than my non-Hashi's counterparts.

Dr. Jack Kruse (controversial and brilliant Neurosurgeon) has a theory possibly explaining dehydration in Hashi's patients: he suggests that EMFs affect the autoimmune patient's cells more deeply, leaving the cell with more heat within and therefore, more easily dehydrated. (www.jackkruse.com)

Ergo, we need water, even sometimes when we don't feel like it.

I do the alkaline water thing and buy my water at the Water Brewery in town. Owner, Einer Haver, (www.thewaterbrewery.com) does what I think is a great job of not only cleaning water of the offending chloride and fluorides, but he revitalizes the water by running it in patterns that mimic the way water runs in the earth. Then, he adds liquid trace minerals back into the water.

When I drink a glass of his water, I actually feel my thirst satisfied. No dry tongue.

Weird, right?

Pimp Your Water

Getting all our water in is essential but isn't always easy. So, I'm going to share some of my little tips, in case you're in a water rut.

Dandelion Tea: sometimes, I go through a dandelion tea stint, like I'm in right now – where I'll brew up a batch, add some honey and lemon, and throw it over ice in a big mason jar and toss in a straw.

It makes me feel home-y like one of those women who sew up their kids' jeans when they get a hole in them. Or like someone who would sit on a front porch and look at the Lands End catalog. Yeah, I'm a wanna-be that kind of person, but mostly am not. I'm the kind of person who accidently leaves the honey out, and then, the ants find it and then, I want to move to another country.

So, drinking tea out of a mason jar feels like I'm Living the Dream.

Apple Cider Vinegar: sometimes I'll put Bragg's ACV in my water. I'll throw that in to a big mason jar to do something healing for my digestion and the alkalinity in my body. The state of our body's ph is either alkaline, neutral or acidic. We're looking to be neutral-to-slightly alkaline, because less gunky stuff happens and more good stuff happens inside of us when our body is out of an acidic state (look at all that amazing science right there – you heard it here first, folks.)

Malic acid (the acid you'd find in apples) becomes alkaline in our system. Pretty nifty. There's a fabulous book by the Bragg's people of all the good uses for ACV, totally worth the shekels.

Liquids Make the World Go 'Round

And, drumroll for my all-time fav:

Lemon: the juice from lemons is excellent for your system. It's great for your digestion and in my Italian culture, folks would start off the day with warm water with lemon to keep things 'regular', if you know what I mean.

And yes, lemon, though it is an acid, is similar to malic acid in that it leaves the result of greater alkalinity in your body. It's because most of the fruit's components are alkaline and the acid component is the weaker thing, leaving you with the benefit of an alkaline experience.

Other things I add to water to keep me from being bored:

- Orange
- Lime
- Cucumber slices
- A splash of unsweetened cherry juice (really good for the gall bladder)

If I get bored and don't drink water, I act like a goober – all outside of myself and feeling funky. Finding some creative ways to get the liquids in, keeps me from getting bored and underhydrated.

Cuckoo for Coconuts

When I've been dizzy and under-hydrated, I've turned to real coconut water.

Like from a *real* coconut.

You're Not Crazy and You're Not Alone

Which is a really foreign animal when you were raised in the North East. Then, I moved to California, which is a great place to explore natural remedies...

Like coconuts.

Coconuts are an amazing remedy – the water, the meat, the milk, and the oil.

But before studying deeper into their healing values, there were only three things I knew about coconuts before I ever consumed them:

1. They often fell from a tree and clonked Gilligan on the head and the most inopportune moments. Poor Gilligan.

2. Their electrolyte make up is very close to the human body's electrolyte make up, and coconut water was used, during war times, as an IV for dehydration as well as transfusions in place of plasma.

3. They're super good for the thyroid and metabolism.

That was all I knew.

But there's a TON of more good stuff they offer.

(Check this out: www.coconutresearchcenter.org)

For me, the real challenge was opening one up. While I'm already an expert at staring at supplements, I had a sincere desire to actually eat and drink from the inside of a real, live coconut.

Liquids Make the World Go 'Round

I learned to open a young Thai coconut (the naked white one, not the Gilligan's Island brown, hairy one) by watching YouTube.

I love YouTube.

Most of the time.

But then, there are times when you're watching something serious like the video on radiation leaks and then, in like three clicks of related subjects, they're giving you porn videos. I'm like, "Hmmm ... "

That's why, when my kids ask if they can hang out on You Tube to watch Pokemon, I say, "No" because I know that Pokemon, three clicks later is going to turn into something like "Poking Man" or something else that's gross.

What *is* it YouTube? Why do you make it that *all roads lead to porn* on your page?

Maybe they'll answer me if someone from the YouTube Company has Hashimoto's and reads my book.

"Hi, person from YouTube. Welcome. Can we chat?"

But I digress...

Back to me and the coconuts (which now sounds completely inappropriate in light of what I've just shared.)

It was a comical sight to behold: me, in the kitchen, with protective eye goggles on my face, a hammer in one hand and a screwdriver in the other standing over an object that is about the size of a small bowling ball and just slightly harder than a diamond, while I'm watching a YouTube video on 'How to Open a Coconut.'

(A video, which I should subtitle, 'Because you really can't save the liquid from the inside of a coconut after you've dropped it onto your concrete patio from the second story window of your house.' True story, btw, and as you guessed, a personal experience. But still – that's a pretty long subtitle.)

Anyway, after several tries, I got one open AND was actually able to collect enough of the water to drink. God, I love it. It's great for under-hydration with all those electrolytes in it and it's very refreshing. You can buy a case at your local Asian market for much cheaper than you can at your health food store. They're the same ones. I've checked.

And even though they are irradiated coming into our country, health coach, Arnoux Goran (www.thmastery.com) had tests done to determine if the radiation affected the enzymatic integrity of the fruit. The result? The enzymes and electrolytes are still in tact after they are irradiated. The shell on a coconut is an amazing source of protection.

Hmmm....Maybe we should all be walking around wearing coconut shell clothing since Fukishima.

Hmm....

Sounds like a YouTube video in the making.

But I digress...

Liquids Make the World Go 'Round

Again.

Anyway.

Coconut water from a fresh coconut is my first choice. I'll use cans of coconut water for my smoothies sometimes. It's pretty good but just not my all-time fave -- but in a pinch, I'm good. If drinking it from a can, I highly recommend that you chill it first. Warm cans of coconut water sometimes reminds me of cat pee, sorry to say. Not all, just some – coconut water that is, not cats. It's not like I go around smelling the pee of different cats.

That would be gross.

Wow. Okay, stay on task, Stace...

Juicing

So, one of my last favorite ways to get my liquids in is juicing.

I luh-ove juicing.

Wait, let me clarify – I love the benefits of juicing and all the yummy tasting combos that you can get in a juice. I don't however, love cleaning my juicer. But it is one of those things in life where the benefits FAR outweigh the inconvenience.

My favorite combo is a couple of carrots, a few stalks of celery, 1/3 of a beet, some green apple, half a lemon (without the skin but WITH as much of the pith as you can. I love that word, *pith*), a bunch of chard and a bit of ginger. Oh. My. Yum.

You're Not Crazy and You're Not Alone

One of my easy summer ways to hydrate is a cucumber and some watermelon. Then, I take the bits that I would throw in my compost pile (if I had a compost pile) and I put it on my face. So, I drink the juice, put the bits on my face for twenty minutes and my skin is super groovy.

The micronutrients from juicing are quickly available to your system because there's very little fiber to slow down the absorption of the nutritious liquid. That makes it super hydrating.

And if you're one of the 12 people in the world who haven't yet watched Joe Cross' juicing journey on "Fat, Sick and Nearly Dead" let me HIGHLY recommend this encouraging film to you: www.fatsickandnearlydead.com.

So, yeah. That's my dealio with the water-o. Some of the creative ways I get it in and a few other options to boot.

The Power of a Blessing

Sometimes, I'll hand my boys a glass of water or a juice or something and I'll tell them to put their hands around the glass and to bless it. Someone taught me years ago that we can charge our water by holding the glass in our hands and blessing it.

Super cool idea.

Then, not long after, I read about the amazing Dr. Masuru Emoto who did a test on water molecules. Have you heard of him? If you haven't, go to YouTube and check out his awe-inspiring videos.

Liquids Make the World Go 'Round

Dr. Emoto wrote words on a piece of paper, words like 'Love' and 'Beauty', and placed them on the glass of water. Then, he put the molecules under a microscope. The molecules became something so absolutely divine and otherworldly. The molecular structure was gorgeous! It made me think of how I imagined Narnia to be when I read the book as a child – all crystalline and stunning.

But when he placed the words 'Fear' or 'Hate' and other negative words on a piece of paper affixed to the glass of water, the molecules under the microscope were ugly and even, dare I say demonic looking.

When we look at the universe in its grandest or smallest parts, sometimes we are so fixated on the power we have to see it that we forget the power we have to affect it.

Our words matter.
Our thoughts about ourselves matter.
The way we bless or curse ourselves, matters.

Remember the whole point of this thing – it's not really about the Hashimoto's – it's that Hashimoto's is the vehicle we have to get back in touch with loving ourselves.

Our body, mind and spirit are a vast universe, housed inside of our flesh, comprised of the smallest cells and atoms that make up our being.

Use your words to bless you.
Recognize the thoughts you have and where they are not a blessing to you.

You're Not Crazy and You're Not Alone

In my book "Bloom Beautiful" I have a quote:

You know how the saying goes, 'The truth shall set you free.'
So, here's the deal
If you're making assessments of yourself:

'I'm unworthy.'
'I'm unlovable.'
'I'm undeserving.'

And you're not wildly freed by those thoughts
Then, it's gotta be
That they're

Just
Not
True.

Maybe you're thinking right now: wait a minute. Wasn't this chapter about liquids?

And the answer is: yes.

But you know what it's really about?

It's about taking care of yourself.
And ultimately that shows up in the smallest and simplest of ways.

Including something like, oh, I don't know ... having a glass of water, perhaps?

Liquids Make the World Go 'Round

Did you say, a glass of water? Why! That's a fabulous idea.

Why don't you make mine
A double.

Cheers!

Chapter 8

Bite-Size Exercise and Queen-Size Pantyhose

I was an athletic kid.

Raised in the Northeast, my summers would be spent out playing from after breakfast until my mom called my sisters and me in for lunch. And then, we'd be out again, riding bikes, climbing trees, running down uneven sidewalks and stubbing our toes until we were called in for dinner.

The winters were spent cheerleading, doing gymnastics and roller-skating around the basement to the tunes of Bay City Rollers and Donna Summer.

And in the Fall and Spring I played in sports. Whether it was boys' baseball (yes, I was the only girl) or girls' softball, more cheerleading, and swimming. And then, in between all that – God, I'm about to date myself – the Jane Fonda workouts on tape that I'd play on my Sony Walkman – the cassette version.

I also loved to take long walks. It was how I dealt with the angst of my teenage years, or my imperfect home life or whatever was the internal crisis du jour. I would take off for miles and hours at a time.

You're Not Crazy and You're Not Alone

So, when I started gaining weight as an adult, and not realizing it was Hashimoto's Hypothyroidism, I got a personal trainer. We worked out, and I mean hard, despite my exhaustion. I wrote down every drop of food that hit my lips. Not only was I not losing, which was perplexing and insulting enough, but I was gaining anywhere between 10-15 pounds a month.

That's up a dress size to a size and a half every month, in dog years.

Within about 10 months, I was up 100 lbs and wearing a size 28/3x, tent moo-moo sized clothes after having been a sexy, curvy size 10.

Now, I'm not sure why they put big flowers or horizontal stripes on big clothes. They might as well come with an announcement, 'On the chance you didn't see how ginormous I am at 270 lbs., this is EXACTLY how big my ass is ...' I mean really, why don't they just stick a measuring tape along your backside and an arrow pointing in the direction of your butt.

Which reminds me of a funny story, speaking of stuff on your backside....

So, while I was increasing in size, I was working at a hotel/fine-dining restaurant where my husband I would perform music. He would play sax, I would play piano and we'd both sing. People loved us and we had a good time traveling around the country doing our music.

It was our routine that I'd go in first to start an hour of solo instrumental music, while my husband hung out in the hotel room, and then, joined me with his sax on the second set.

We were getting ready one night. I was in the hotel room, opening my new pair of Queen-size pantyhose (oh God, remember those? Do they even still MAKE pantyhose? Do people even still *wear* them??). I threw the wrapper on the chair and walked around the room. I was watching some show, chatting with Rock while I was hopping and doing the 'Putting on my pantyhose' dance until the elastic was snug around my waist. I put on my black slacks and black top, sat down to put on my shoes, grabbed my music bag, and kissed the man goodbye.

I walked into the dining room, which was dark except for low lighting and the flickering candlelight on tables. It was filled with well-dressed couples and soft-spoken servers tending to the needs of the already-filled room.

As my custom, I would walk around and greet the regulars at the tables, introduce myself and ask for any requests. After about 10-15 minutes of moving about the room and chatting with folks, I walked the expanse of the dance floor on my way to the stage, past the bar and in front of all the people in the restaurant.

One of my friends, Lorri, who had a strong Texas accent was working that night. She had the strangest look on her face, came right up to me and said in a not-too-soft voice, "What the hell is this?" reached around and pulled off of my backside the pantyhose outer cardboard envelope. The opening flap had stuck to my butt when I had sat down to put on my shoes, creating a sort of sign with the pantyhose packaging which was all white, except for the big, purple cursive lettering announcing, 'QUEEN SIZE' for all the world to see.

You're Not Crazy and You're Not Alone

Oh. My. Lord.

Looking back, it's hilarious in that, 'Oh noooooo … tell me that really didn't happen … ' kind of way that makes your eyes bug out when you hear about it.

But, back then? Then, I wanted to fall into a big, gaping hole in the ground. See, I was still trying to hold my falling-apart life, together. It hadn't fully collapsed and I hadn't found my sense of humor yet.

But I digress…

Back to exercise. So, no matter what I did, how much cardio I ran, and how many weights I lifted – no matter how much of the stationary bike I rode or how many aerobics classes I took, I still. gained. weight.

Why?

I had heard years ago about how the mitochondria (the part of our cells that break down nutrients and make chemical energy for our body) in autoimmune patients functions differently when we exercise. Dr. Brett Jacques, a fabulous Naturopath and a Hashimoto's patient himself explains why:

"Hashimoto's patients have severe mitochondrial dysfunction and poor ATP generation (how the body moves energy to the cells) so they are not able to, and should not exercise much, if at all. Based on labs and patient presentation, I recommend walking and weights for my Hashi's patients.

Bite-Size Exercise and Queen-Size Pantyhose

By walking I mean sauntering at the beach barefoot in the sand 2-4 times per week for 10-30 minutes. The weight training I recommend is very basic and limited in time and frequency. It isn't a pink dumbbell workout, I want them to strength train with a few reps, few sets and plenty of rest between sets. They should be in and out of the gym in 15-20 minutes, twice a week."

I have often heard anecdotes over the years from frustrated former marathoners or frustrated hard-core exercise enthusiasts that they didn't have energy anymore and they were gaining weight. I wasn't the only one. The common theme? Hashimoto's.

Bob Dirgo, author of How I Reversed My Hashimoto's Thyroiditis Hypothyroidism, talked about how he would run a high amount of miles a day and just couldn't anymore once he had Hashimoto's. He said, "Intense levels of exercise, such as experienced with training for and participating in marathons, puts a strain on the body. This type of exertion has been show to weaken the immune system making the body susceptible to immune system related disorders."

So, even though exercise is good (in general), when you're in a Hashimoto's state, the body perceives it as a stress instead of a benefit.

I was personally experiencing the reality of that.

The more I exercised, the more my body shut down.

At some point we figured out I had hypothyroidism and I started on Synthroid. The doctor said, "Oh, you're going to lose this extra weight in three months!" I kept eating in my Fettuccine Alfredo

Vegetarian, not-really-healthy way) and swam 50 laps several times a week despite being in excruciating pain. Three months later, I had gained 30 more pounds. I looked like I had eaten myself.

A different approach was required for this different time.

My thyroid was a swollen mess and I was in physical pain. Synthroid (the synthetic thyroid med) and I didn't get along. I was switched to Levoxyl (a different synthetic med). Come to find out that Synthroid has gluten in it. Not my friend, my friend. With a remedy like that, who needs an enemy? Anyway...

At a certain point, an Orange Cone, disguised as an endocrinologist, told me he was tired of messing around with my thyroid and wanted to cut it out. When I asked him what the complications were he said, "Well, yours is enlarged in the back and it's all wrapped around the vocal cord nerve. So, it's possible we *could* nick the nerve and your voice could either change or worst case, it could be paralyzed for life."

I stared at him, waiting for him to say, "Just kidding!" and then, tell me the real story, but he was serious.

I said, "Dr. Orange Cone, you know I'm a singer and a speaker. That's my career...is there any other option available to me?" He snorted, mocking me and said, "Hmph ... *God.*" He laughed.

And right before I left he made mention of me walking for at least 5 minutes a day. I tucked that away in my cap.

So, I left his office, made an appointment with the surgeon, not for surgery, but just to gather info. I went home to pray about this thyroid thing. "God, give me Wisdom."

I went to the surgeon. Like I said, I didn't want to have my thyroid out. I didn't plan to have my thyroid out. It just wasn't *peace* to me. My prayer had included being open to hear what Wisdom this guy would have for me. He was one of the best surgeons in the area and was known around the world. I didn't know if he'd have Wisdom or if he'd be an Orange Cone – I didn't know. I was just following a mix of inspiration and fear.

It was a fancy, shmancy office in Newport Beach, California where people who are already skinny and pretty enough, would sit and wait for their appointment to be skinnier and prettier via scalpel.

Here I was, all 270 pounds of me, looking like I could eat a skinny person or two for lunch and still have room for dessert, standing there waiting to be seen.

I was standing because I couldn't sit in the chairs that had arms on them. The other women were sitting there, in their little doll clothes with room for at least three of their skinny friends to sit beside them. I, on the other hand, looked longingly at the chairs. In my fantasy world, I imagined being able to sit down in an armchair and actually be able to stand up again without the damn thing being stuck to my ass.

I went into the surgeon's office. It smelled of money. The doctor was overweight under his white coat, about 55, but looked older with his tousled grey hair, and shook my hand like I was contagious.

You're Not Crazy and You're Not Alone

He barely looked at me. I understood. I barely wanted to look at me. I was painfully obese, my hair had turned from blonde to orange, my eyebrows were half missing like Mr. Spock (only not as cool) and my skin was a mess. It was covered with scabbed-over yeast patches called Seborrheic Dermatitis. It was lovely. Oh, and as you can imagine, my energy was very low and I was depressed. If I could have run away to another country and left my body behind, I would have gladly done that.

The doctor studied my labs, took my stats, felt my thyroid, and started writing notes.

I told him my thyroid had been so swollen that I was choking on food when I ate. He nodded. I told him I sang and spoke for a living, and even though I was on hiatus from that for a while, I was concerned about changes in my voice with a surgery. He grunted something indistinguishable and wrote more notes.

When he finally spoke, the first thing he asked was, "Can you go three months without eating solid food?" I had already been avoiding solids anyway, out of fear of choking to death.

"Yes. I can do that."

When he asked me about exercise, I told him I was on hiatus from that, too but that Dr. Orange Cone told me to walk 5 minutes a day. He asked, "Can you do that?"

I was in pain all over my body and in such a fragile state, despite my large wall-like appearance, but I nodded, "Yes."

After a few more notes and a measurement around my neck, he

walked over to me.

"I don't want to do surgery on you, Mrs. Robbins. Sometimes, the body goes in cycles. I want to see if you can cycle out of this in the next few months. If not, we'll talk about surgery but for now, that is my recommendation."

I sighed huge relief. Dr. Not-An-Orange Cone

And I left.

The next day, even though I felt like I was dying from all the pains in my body as well as the exhaustion and inner stress, my husband drove me down to the beach.

Gone were the days of riding bikes and hearty swims or climbing trees. I was so sick, I could barely climb in and out of the car. It took 15 minutes to get to the beach, and 15 minutes back for a 5-minute walk in between.

We did that every day.

Five minutes of walking.

My diet was mostly comprised of fatty soups that I'd buy at the grocery store – either hot from the deli section or from a can heated up and then blended. Also, there were the ice cream shakes and smoothies several times a day, which in retrospect were almost completely gluten-free, how interesting …

And within three to four months of gentle exercise and doing the liquid diet, I had lost 70 pounds.

You're Not Crazy and You're Not Alone

(Now, I'm not necessarily advocating you do my food or exercise program. I am much more thoughtful about eating whole, fresh foods since then. I'm an ingredient detective, opting for organic veggies/fruits, and grass fed meats whenever possible. I'm just telling you my story of what I did back then.)

The walking turned into 7 minutes. Then, 10. And eventually 20. Within about six months, I was up to 30 minutes a day.

I wasn't fast. I didn't break a sweat. But I did create a new habit and lifestyle that included exercise in a way that was friendly to my body and my healing.

Thirteen years later, I still walk about 45- 60 minutes, five days a week.

Sometimes when I'm going through a Hashi's flare, my walk is 10 minutes long and I do that a few times a day. Some days, I just bag it. Because I'm listening for the wisdom of whether rest is what I need more than a walk. But the point is that it's so much a part of my life again. This time, in a non-stressful way.

My dear friends, who see that I still have weight to lose, are always trying to drag me to their gym, or to boot camp, or Crossfit.

I'm like, "Thank you! But the last time I did a boot camp, I had black spots in front of my eyes for 10 days and it took two months to heal from all the pain."

Even though, those programs work for them, I can't, and *will not* let myself get pressured into thinking that they work for me.

Bite-Size Exercise and Queen-Size Pantyhose

Exercise is not a one-size-fits-all proposition. Especially when you have an autoimmune dis-ease.

I have friends with Hashimoto's who still run, and that feels good for them. I have a guy friend with Hashimoto's who said, "Screw the gentle exercise, I'm not letting anything stop me!" and he works out, balls-to-the-wall hard and swears by it. I'm so happy for him.

For my hard-core work-out friends, I tell them, "I used to bench press my weight when I was 135 lbs. Now, I have two hernias and need my boys lift the gallon of milk for me."

I'm kidding, of course, I lift the gallon of milk but the point is this: I know me. I know what works and does the least amount of harm. Respecting my adrenal glands matters more to me than the size of my thighs.

I'm open to being enlightened to the next phase of exercise that I can add. I'd love to lose these under arm flaps that wiggle as I wave (by the way, that extra 'baggage' under there is a common symptom of hypothyroidism and adrenal fatigue.) I used to call them my 'lunch lady arms' but I try not to talk about myself that way anymore. I work on being kinder to me.

If I don't ever berate or put down my children and expect them to thrive, why I do that to myself?

(Answer: well, because...honestly? I think I have this shadowy alter ego who wants to have a second career as a sassy, snarky comedienne. I'm pretty funny and have about 30 ways I can make fun of my butt alone. But, there's this little thing that niggles in me that says, "Hey! Be kind to you!" If I wouldn't say it to my kid, and I wouldn't let them say it to another kid, then, why am I talking about myself this way?

Please hear me, I'm not trying to make a religion out of this, 'Thou shall not use those words!' because that's its own bondage of performance and perfectionism. Nothankyouverymuch. But I'm just exploring how powerful our thoughts and words are. That awareness is helping me to shift how I think and what I say. Sometimes that means, I give up getting a laugh, for the sake of speaking *life* over myself.)

Back to exercising …

I like the walking I do, and I have a dream of running on the beach – but not at any cost.

Because I'm not living in a movie, I'm living in my life. I have had to let go of the romantic notions of what looks good, just because I saw it on a film with star-crossed lovers running on the beach. I'll trade that for the reality-based endeavors of what is healthy and feels good.

I occasionally do gentle weights or one of those resistance bands. I've done yoga and really, really enjoy that and keep threatening to do more. But the point is this:

Be kind to yourself.
Exercise should be a blessing…
To your body.
And your mind.
And your spirit.

Bite-Size Exercise and Queen-Size Pantyhose

And if your body isn't responding to one way of exercising, try another.

If you're used to muscling your way through your workout routine the same way you muscle your way through life, maybe it's time to try a new way.

A kinder way.
A gentler way.

And if you're not doing anything because you're being perfectionistic or feeling hopeless, check in with your health care professional and find out if it's safe for you to do something. You may find out as I did, that the best remedy, not only for the perfectionism and hopelessness, but for your body, is to take a small walk.

Exercise is about getting your body moving, but it does so much more than that: it clears the cobwebs away in your brain, it makes those happy chemicals, the endorphins, come out and play. It shifts your breathing from shallow to deep.

This isn't about competing.
Or doing it like your neighbor.
Or like you used to.

This isn't a movie.
This is your life.

Part of loving yourself is about connecting to this body that you have been over-focused on and yet, neglecting all at the same time.

You're Not Crazy and You're Not Alone

Your body has done a lot for you all these years and it's been waving the little white flag telling you that it needs some focused attention. This is your moment in time to give it a little TLC. Even just for five little minutes a day.

I'm saying this with all love and sincerity:

Go take a hike.

Just make it a gentle one.

Chapter 9

Minerals, Yurts, and Men Who Groan

I really didn't have a fuller grasp about the importance of minerals until I was lying on a table in a chiropractor's office, next to a guy who was making the most distracting, groaning noises during an adjustment.

Though there was not one sexual thing going on, he sounded like he was rehearsing for his part in a porn flick.

As open and woo-woo as I am about stuff – and I know the guy was just releasing tension, because I've heard men and women do those vocal exhales all the time in yoga classes or meditation clinics – that day, it was just bugging me. And I didn't want to spend my 45 minutes with my butt clenched so, I almost asked Dr. Silvana, one of my amazing Chiropractors, if I could switch from the room with four tables into the private room, instead.

But then, I thought, 'Wait, Stacey. Sometimes when people are extremely irritating, they have an extreme gift to give to you.'

So, I breathed deeply and tried to go to my happy place. Well, not as happy as his place apparently, but my own, rather-reserved-by-comparison 'happy place.'

You're Not Crazy and You're Not Alone

Silvana walked up to my table, "Stacey, you are just looking great! You're losing weight!"

I was face down and smiling through that little hole in the table, "I know! Isn't it cool? I'm so excited! And look at my feet, too!" I lifted them up so she could peek. "The cracks are going away."

Seriously, you've never seen someone as excited about smooth feet as I was. I had tried just about every lotion, cream, and foot spa treatment but to no avail – the cracks that happen around the edges of the feet, from having an autoimmune issue, are an inside-out job. My insides were healing and it was showing up on my feet!

So Mr. Groany-Man from the table next to me asks, "What are you doing to make that happen? Are you taking something?"

"Yes. Actually, I am." I thought for a second about where to start, "I started taking one new thing, and it's the only thing I'm taking, other than my thyroid medicine, come to think of it…"

I turned on my side so Silvana could adjust my atlas while I kept telling the story.

"Three months ago, I had started taking this BioLumina Spirulina and I have been feeling so good on it! My heels had been all cracked and bleeding for years from my thyroid. Six weeks after taking this BioLumina, my husband noticed that my feet had new skin on them." I paused and went on, "Then, I started losing weight, like really losing weight. I've lost 25 lbs in six weeks."

"Oh yes," He said, "Spirulina is an incredible food source and it's rich with minerals. Your body can't recover, your skin can't heal and you can't lose weight until you have the proper minerals in your system. Spirulina is very re-mineralizing."

Silvana said, "Stacey, this is John -- he's a brilliant guy. Been a nutritionist for over 30 years. This man knows his stuff."

Wow. What a gift.

John said to me, "I've never heard of BioLumina, though. Where do you get it?"

I told him, "Me. I am so convinced about this, that I started selling it."

I started telling him the story about how it came my way.

And trust me (I'm talking to you reading right now, not to John) while I know this sounds like one ginormous commercial to "Come buy BioLumina – from me!" you know me by now, there's more to this story and I want you to hear how serendipitous it was, because it will encourage you in how it all played out.

Here's the story:

You know how some days you're just sitting on your computer floating around the Internet? You may start of doing a Google search for a way to do your own at-home-manicure, and then, an hour later you end up on YouTube watching a video on the 40-year history of radiation detonations in the world.

Yeah, so that's pretty much what happened to me.

You're Not Crazy and You're Not Alone

I ended up watching this compelling YouTube video called "Nuclear Detonation Timeline 1945-1998" and was shocked at all the radiation explosions, exposures, tests and leaks that have happened around the world and especially so many close to me in California.

By the way, this was prior to the Fukishima nuclear disaster.

After watching the video, I was stunned. I put my computer aside, sat cross-legged on my couch and placed my hand over my thyroid, "God. Please help me. Please give me a solution to protect our thyroids from radiation. And especially to protect our children from radiation. Please lead me to Wisdom."

I was heavy-hearted because I know how affected thyroids are from radiation. And I know, too well, the lasting effect of having one of these master glands so deeply compromised.

I didn't want any further damage to me and I didn't want my children --- and the children of the generations -- to be dealing with a compromised thyroid. I didn't want their moods and metabolism affected or their immune systems suppressed. I didn't want them or their future spouses to deal with infertility issues or have a higher likelihood of in utero deformities.

Turning my heavy-hearted concerns into a prayerful meditation allowed me to leave the burden at the door of the Divine.

It was about three months later my friend, Irene, and I drove up for some healing treatments in Northern California. We found ourselves sitting outside of a yurt, which was surrounded by an earthy, rustic community of homes – quiet and inspiring in the woods – waiting our turn for a treatment.

When Irene went in to the yurt for her treatment, one of the own-ers of the houses came out to her garden and started chatting with me.

I instantly liked her. She was warm and friendly, good-natured and seemed so comfortable with herself. I couldn't tell how old she was but I could tell that in her youth she had spent a good amount of time in the sun. Without a stitch of make up on you could see the freckles that had come over time. I was so touched by the warmth in her eyes and her beautiful speaking voice.

Her name was Lyndia. We got to chatting and she asked what I did, "Well, I'm on a healing journey right now, after a few bumpy years – so, thank you for letting your yurt be used for our heal-ing." She nodded, "Of course, you're welcome."

I told her I was a writer, a speaker, a health advocate and a coun-selor of sorts.

"What do you do, Lyndia?"

She smiled, "Well, I've done many things in my life, mostly re-lated to health and spirituality. My husband, Lance, and I have a product that we care for and sell that helps people, especially children to be protected from the effects of radiation."

Now, it was my turn to smile.

At no point in my introduction had I mentioned my prayer a few months back about radiation. At no point did I tell her that private heart's desire to protect children.

I asked her the name of the product and the name of her company.

The company is New Phoenix Rising. As soon as I heard the name, I knew I was supposed to be connected to her.

It might sound crazy -- you're probably already used to me by now -- but I saw this as so serendipitous. Not just because of my prayer and her answer. But because my name 'Stacey' means 'Like a phoenix, rising from the ashes.' And my astrological sign, in its highest calling means 'like a phoenix rising.'

So, at the risk of sounding kooky, I felt like there were a lot of points of connection to me with Lyndia and Lance, and for me to learn more about this product.

The next day, we chatted more about my life and hers. She made me a BioLumina smoothie before we hit the road. It was delicious.

When I came back home to my husband, I told him the story. He was standing in the kitchen staring at me. I get stared at a lot. "You hate spirulina, Stacey."

"I do?"

"Oh god, don't you remember? Someone told you to take it years ago. You bought this big thing, it tasted like dirt and you threw out the whole package."

I said, "Well, I don't remember that, but I believe you. Maybe this product is different."

And it was. I bought it, loved it, actually TOOK it (you know me and my penchant for buying things and then, staring at them on the counter. Not with this one. I was faithful.) and gave it to our family. I started noticing differences in my health.

Point is: since I was still on this learning curve with spirulina, I didn't know the mineral component until I was on the table next to John, the Groaner.

Then, I looked up the importance of minerals in our body: I found this blurb on the Divine Health website of my friend Lydia Shatney's (not to be confused with Lyndia Leonard of BioLumina – dear Lord, out of all the chapters I have in this book, it's *this* one that I put both Lyndia AND Lydia's name in the same sentence ...)

"Minerals are basically the spark plugs of life, or keystones to our health. Minerals are the catalysts that keep our 'battery' going and hold its 'charge.' Minerals compose about 4% of the human body. We cannot produce minerals within our bodies, so we must obtain them through our food. They ultimately come from the earth. Good soil is 45% minerals, yet our soils today are quite lacking due to synthetic fertilizers, mono-cropping and more. In the US our soils contain 86% less minerals than they did 100 years ago (based on a study done in 1992)."

- Minerals act as cofactors for enzyme reactions. Enzymes don't work without minerals. All cells require enzymes to work & function. They give us our vitality.
- They maintain the pH balance within the body.

- Minerals actually facilitate the transfer of nutrients across cell membranes.
- They maintain proper nerve conduction.
- Minerals help to contract and relax muscles.
- They help to regulate our bodies tissue growth.
- Minerals provide structural and functional support for the body.

(Lydia Joy Shatney, certified Nutritional Therapy Practitioner http://divinehealthfromtheinsideout.com/2012/05/the-role-of-minerals-in-the-body/)

Minerals are essential for our body's health and healing. Whether you get them from BioLumina, bone broth, ground pastured egg shells (yes, people do that, so rich in Calcium) or another source you trust and love, it's important you look into them because here's the deal: if minerals are a significant part of our health then, being deficient in them can be a significant part of our unhealth, especially with Hashimoto's.

So grateful for the gift of Lyndia and BioLumina spirulina and the gift of John, lying next to me that day at my doctor's appointment.

Sometimes the best gifts come at unexpected times and unexpected places – like in a prayer on the couch in the middle of the night, or in a garden by a yurt in the middle of the Redwoods, or on a table in the middle of a chiropractic appointment...

With a very strange man
groaning next to you.

Chapter 10

Labels, Labels, Everywhere...

It makes me kind of crazy that we've become a world full of people who are labeled. By our race, religion, relationships, resources, real-estate and so much more.

We're fraught with acronyms and labels that define, never thinking about how they might limit us.

I had my experience with that, first-hand, in my marriage.

(BTW, this approaching TMI moment is something my husband and I used to speak about publicly and counseled other folks in so, don't lose your breath. It's not a secret and I'm not betraying anything.)

When Rock and I got married, I didn't know he had an issue with pornography. It was something I found out about six months into our marriage that he had carried from his teen years. All the expected feelings followed: rejection, betrayal, embarrassment, disappointment ... on both our parts.

I wanted him to be over and done with it, like yesterday, but it was a process of seven years. Every day is long when you're living in a situation with the mistress of a compulsive habit (we don't call it an 'addiction' in our house). Those seven years seemed like a lifetime when we were going through them, but seem like a blip on the screen now, after 25 years of marriage.

We tried religious counseling and secular counseling but it wasn't like it is these days, with tons of resources to help a couple through this. This was almost 25 years ago and there wasn't a lot of help out there. At least not that we found.

One of the options was to attend SA: Sexaholics Anonymous. While I'm a believer in some of the elements of the 12-step process, I honestly had an issue with the whole "Hi, my name is_____and I'm a whatever-aholic."

So, I shared my thoughts with Rock and asked him, "Are you going to stand up and say that when you introduce yourself?" He said, "I don't know. Why?"

I shook my head in an unconvinced way and let him know where I was at, "Honey, I don't think that slapping a label on you is going to free you from this. In fact, I think just the opposite: I think that you saying that sentence ends up being a 'sentence'.

Why put yourself in the prison of some label? And beside, why would you want people to know that as part of your identity? Is that what you want people to thinking of when they see you: 'Oh, look! There's Rocky, the Pornaholic.'"

He leaned against the wall and nodded for me to keep going. "Look, pornography is not who you are, it's what you're doing right now to cope with pain. And you can change what you do in a New York minute so, why imprison yourself in that label?"

Labels, Labels Everywhere...

He thought about it. Before he left for the meeting, I said something that clicked with me – but I wasn't sure if it clicked with him.

"You are *not* what you do. It's a habit and it has consequences. But if you label yourself that way, you become a victim to that label. If you're going to have any kind of label over you, it should be Love because that's who you are. That's who you were created to be and that's never going to change."

I had never said that before. It just kind of came out of my mouth. I didn't know, that 20 years after that, I was going to have a huge revelation about how we are all created from Love ...

I feel that way about any label, including Hashimoto's. Even though it is so liberating to have had a diagnosis other than 'anxiety', I don't want to be defined by Hashimoto's or limit myself because of it. Yes, of course, my life has required that I make some significant changes, and understanding more about this dis-ease is so helpful.

God, yes!

And yes, it's been a catalyst for me to discover how I have let my life go by without truly caring for myself. I've been learning a lot about how to love myself through this diagnosis of Hashimoto's.

I am so grateful for the clarity.

But I am not my label, or my diagnosis. Just like someone walking around with cancer doesn't say, "I am cancer." Or someone with bursitis doesn't say, "I am bursitis."

You're Not Crazy and You're Not Alone

Being diagnosed _with_ something and being diagnosed _as_ something are two different things.

There's a difference between identifying something _in_ your life and being identified _by_ it.

I don't want to confuse the two because I want to live as free a life as possible. And I'm aware that our words can either be stepping stones of freedom that we set along our path, or they can be the bars on the prison that we create for ourselves.

Sometimes we enjoy being the victim who has the label. We get the benefit of attention or we get the justification for being out of sorts, or we get the validation that yes, life hurt us and we're sad.

Sometimes it's a control thing: we make people revolve their unhealthy lives around our unhealthy life. It's the only way we know love to function so, we perpetuate the patterns that we learned even when they're not healthy.

We hold people hostage to our label and call it 'our dis-ease.' They can't go anywhere or do anything because we can't. They can't be productive or happy because we're not. And if they do actually get to go out, we make them feel guilty so they don't have quite as much fun as they could have.

We become victim terrorists.

But that's coming from fear. All of it. Fear of not being loved for who we are. Fear of not being important without something being wrong with us. Fear of being forgotten so we "stand out" by being needy.

Labels, Labels Everywhere...

It makes sense. Oh, trust me. But it just doesn't ultimately serve us because it's not coming from love.

Love's goal is freedom.

Love wants freedom from any prison that holds us. Fear wants to lock us in and throw the keys out of the window, into the wilderness, never to be found again.

I have a saying in my book, <u>Bloom Beautiful</u>, it says: "Fear won't tell you the truth about Love, but Love will tell you the Truth about Fear. Seek Love."

It's a lesson my kids are learning, too: about the kind of attention we get for different reasons.

Caleb and Seth got enthralled lately with having casts and ace bandages. They saw how their friends at school, who had an injury that warranted a cast, splint, or sling got a lot of attention.

A few weeks ago, my oldest climbed onto a cool swing that someone had fashioned in a canyon near our house. Caleb did a running jump off the hill one too many times. On the last run and jump, his tired arms gave way and he fell, with great velocity from about 15 feet in the air.

I watched him land with a thump, as my heart went from my chest into the pit of my stomach. His wrist and hip took the brunt of the fall. Once it became clear to me that he was essentially 'okay', it also became clear that it was going to take me longer to heal than it took him.

You're Not Crazy and You're Not Alone

On the second day, his wrist still hurt. He asked for an ace bandage. On the third day, it hurt, too, but less. I bought a new bandage to wrap him up.

He was thrilled, not just to have the wrap, but the attention it gave to justify the pain in his wrist, as well as for his gift of story telling that placed him in the center of the circle on the playground at school.

The next day, my youngest got hurt, literally fell off a neighbors big bike and into the bushes. (Enough with the falling, already.) There were thorn scratches bleeding from his face and body. He was sore inside and out. I was learning how to breathe again.

Seth wanted some Band Aids right on his face. And the next day, getting ready for school, Seth wanted more Band Aids on places that had invisible owies. Caleb wanted his wrist wrapped, even though he said he felt better.

I said, "Guys, I'm happy to wrap and package you up because I want those hurting areas to be safe and I want you to feel safe. I do want to say this, though: the best attention you could ever get in life is from your strengths and not your weaknesses or your injuries."

Do you know that by the end of the day, Caleb's wrap was in his lunchbox and Seth's face was Band Aid free?

You know what Caleb said when I asked him why? "Mom, I just couldn't move with this thing on." And Seth said, "I couldn't play kickball with the Band Aids on my face, it was distracting me."

Labels, Labels Everywhere...

I learned so much that day: they knew that freedom and enjoyment of life was more valuable than the attention they could get from being hurt. They chose the greater thing. I want to be like them when I grow up and choose the greater thing.

To say, "I was diagnosed with Hashimoto's" or "I'm on a healing journey with Hashimoto's" is the empowering way I aim to address my relationship with this autoimmune thing.

I don't want it to be the focus of every time I go out for a meal, "Oh I can't eat that because I have an AI." Which then, leads to some explanation about what 'AI' means. And then dinner becomes the Hashimoto's show, starring ME.

Or when the clerk at the store doesn't treat you right, you have to be sure to tell them that you're hot, cranky, sweaty, freezing, sad, whatever ... because you have Hashimoto's.

And every time your husband wants to have sex, Hashimoto's is the excuse.

You think I'm kidding. I'm not. Some of us get our Master's Degree in Manipulation from V.U. -- Victim University.

I'm not saying we can't invite people into our journey, or we can't learn from the diagnosis. And god, you already know by now, I am ALL about honoring where you are at in this healing process.

I'm just talking about not being identified by it and having others be harangued by it.

I think our language both reflects and creates our mindset.

You're Not Crazy and You're Not Alone

My words will tattle on what's already swimming around in my head as well as pave the way for what's coming in my life.

So, if I see myself as a victim, I'm going to use victim words to describe myself. And if I do that, I'm going to be stepping deeper in to a victim mindset.

I'm not superstitious about it. I'm not afraid of saying something the 'wrong' way and then, beating up myself (or others) about how precisely something was stated. I'm not the 'How You Said It' police. I'm simply conscious of our great power and that words can define us by our greatness or our limitations.

I mentioned in the chapter on Liquids about Dr. Emoto and his experiment – the one where he affixed written words to a glass of water. He documented that, depending on the word that was written on a paper, the molecular structure of the waters changed to either something beautiful, or something horrid.

Then, how can we human beings, who are believed to be at least 70-80% water, not be affected by words as well?

I remember when I left my structured religion and people wanted to know, 'So what are you now? Do you call yourself a Christian? A Buddhist? A Hindu? An Agnostic?'

We feel safer with labels. They become handlebars that help us control our experiences with other people. Like, "Oh whew! Now, I know what you are, so now I can relate to you in a certain way."

Labels make it easy.

Labels, Labels Everywhere...

Because they don't require a whole lot from us.

We don't have to trust. We don't have to engage our heart. We don't have to be in the present moment with each other because we've already figured everything out and go on autopilot.

I mean seriously, take a moment and let yourself be swept away by your definitions when you read these labels:

Republican
Democrat
Christian
Muslim
Jew
Immigrant
Minority
Millionaire
Ex-Convict

We slap labels on people and file the person away. And what we do is we start interacting with the label, and our judgments

Instead of the person.

I simply told the folks who asked, "I call myself a 'human being' because that's what I am. That never changes, no matter what church or temple I walk into. And no one's left out. Everyone belongs to this country club called 'Life.'"

That made some of my friends crazy. They wanted to know if I was on their religious team or if I was on the team that was going to hell. If I was on their team they could relax. If I was on another team, they had to "save" me.

They wanted handlebars, and I gave them a unicycle.

As far as Hashimoto's goes: I let the diagnosis give me wisdom about how to care for myself, not how to label myself. I don't 'limit' myself, my time, my energy and my foods; I 'focus' myself, my time, my energy and my foods.

I have always believed in the possibility of being cured or healed. The doctors would tell me that could never happen. Just like they told me I would never have kids. I didn't agree with their 'never'. I was open to a greater possibility. Unless they are God and know all things, they don't know what's possible. I'm living in the possibility of healing or cure.

So, that's my dealio on this whole thing: I don't want to be a victim of a label,, and I don't want to create a prison for myself.

And neither did my husband. When he came home from that meeting over 20 years ago he said, "I didn't want to do it. I just told them, 'Hi. I'm Rocky.' And sat down."

He wanted to be free, more than he wanted to be limited and labeled.

Just like my kids with their bandages.

And me with Hashimoto's.

I'm grateful to know what's going on. And I don't mind making my schedule smaller as I heal, but I do mind making my belief about

Labels, Labels Everywhere...

myself smaller.

I am not less of a person because of this Hashi's thing. What I *have* and who I *am* are two different things.

My goal is to keep that clear and be open to the possibility of all the possible good that exists for me.

Labels are limiting, but Love is full of possibility.

When we start embracing that, we start seeing that
Anything is possible
In Love.

Chapter 11

With a Family Member Like That, Who Needs An Enemy?

Oh lawdy, lawd.

Where do you even begin when it's the people who know you (and say that they love you) who are sometimes the ones who judge you the most?

It's hard enough to be feeling exhausted all the time. To be dealing with one sinus or Urinary Tract infection after another because your immune system is so wiped out. To have brain fog and memory issues, a stomach that gives out at every meal, a deep dark depression, and to be outgrowing your fat clothes faster than anyone can say, "Mother, May I?"

The last thing you need on top of all *that*, is one of your family members or closest friends looking at you with a scrunched up face that screams, *Eww…would you stop already? What the hell is wrong with you? Everybody's tired. Everybody's stressed. I'm inconvenienced by you not feeling well, so could you please snap out of it!*

That sounds harsh but trust me – that's how many with Hashimoto's and other autoimmune dis-eases have been treated, including myself.

It's a heart-aching moment to feel like such a stranger inside your own skin *and* to feel the rejection of the ones you love, pulsing hot with judgment when they're around you.

I understand.

I'm sorry.

You are not crazy
And you are not alone.

I had gone to the Huntington Library in Pasadena with some family members many years back. The grounds were lovely, but I couldn't seem to focus on enjoying them.
I couldn't keep up with the others as we walked the sidewalks to the rose gardens. I needed to sit more often and kept losing my breath. I looked normal. Normal weight. Normal hair and dress. My external hadn't fallen apart yet but my insides had and they were waving a little white flag. I just didn't know why (yet).

My family members sighed exasperated sighs. Rolled their eyes at me for needing to sit on another bench. Called to me to "Come ON already, Stacey." And then, whispered about me behind my back.

They're good, lovely people in general, who happened to be acting like goobers. That's a kind word, trust me. They just didn't get it.

With a Family Member Like That, Who Needs an Enemy

Neither did I.

I felt like such a failure and a disappointment. I thought they were right, that I was ruining their day. That I was a loser.

Then, there were the other extended family members a few years later. The ones who stood back and judged instead of stepping forward. They criticized me and it would come back to me in that lovely telephone game, 'So-and-so said that you should be taking medication, you shouldn't be trying to do this naturally.'

I said, "I *am* taking medication. Something's just not working right."

I wished they would have asked me questions instead of just assuming things about me. People who judge seem allergic to asking questions.

There were others who were upset that I wasn't working and making money like I used to. Instead of them saying, "Wow, Stacey, you've been the breadwinner of the family and honestly, a workaholic for many years, and now you're sick. It's okay for you to rest and heal ..." No, I got one criticism after another.

These were people I loved. Whom I called 'family.' And I believed that somewhere inside of them, they truly loved me...

Maybe.

But I honestly couldn't feel it with how they were acting.

The judgment was harsh and it cut me like a knife.

You're Not Crazy and You're Not Alone

It wasn't from everyone, just a select few people from each side of our families who honestly, had their own issues of unhappiness before I ever entered the scene. But I didn't have that kind of perspective to see that then. At the time, I just felt incredibly rejected and misunderstood and overcome with so many symptoms.

As I got clearer on one diagnoses after another: Hypothyroidism, PCOS (Polycystic Ovarian Syndrome), myalgias, ocular migraines, heart arrhythmias, hiatal hernia and Hashimoto's, and learned what my body was truly going through, I had compassion on myself.

I realized how much my system was compromised and that it was a pretty serious thing. I felt sad that I had discounted myself so much and that I had let people who really could have (should have?) been there for me, discount me, too.

I wanted to go to them and say, "What the fuck were you even thinking being such a fucking asshole to me when I felt like I was dying? Have you no compassion? Don't tell me you love me and then treat me like shit when I truly need some help. Fuck *you*."

I really did. I went through that phase of feeling really angry. It took me about 12 years to finally *feel* angry but, eventually I went through an angry phase.

That anger, hurt, and frustration from the people you believed were going to really be there for you, and weren't, can become one of the greatest gifts you can receive, if you are willing to see an opportunity in everything.

With a Family Member Like That, Who Needs an Enemy

1. You get the opportunity to not be a victim.

Being a victim is a huge temptation when you get an auto-immune diagnosis. You know why? Because honestly – and please listen carefully to this – so many of us had victimized ourselves to get us to the point of this sickness that we finally feel justified in having a legitimate diagnosis. We finally feel justified in sitting down, crying in our soup, and taking time off of life's treadmill, to heal.

It's like a friend of mine who's a super strong and fiercely powerful woman; she was going through hell in her marriage. Being very private, she wouldn't share it with practically anyone. One day, her ankle gave out on her while she was mountain climbing in Colorado. She stayed home from work. She cried all day long. She got to finally tell people how much something was hurting her – only it was her ankle she had made the voice for her breaking heart.

I feel that is a strong possibility for those of us with Hashimoto's. Where we had been so rejected and loathed by either others or ourselves (or both) and then, this visible, tangible diagnosis is revealed and we're finally able to say, 'See! I AM hurting! I DO need love!'

Many of us were sexually, physically or emotionally abused. The abuse I went through as a child left me with a belief that I was unworthy of being treasured, unworthy of being protected, and unworthy of being loved. I believed I was ruined.

Unfortunately, on the heels of that abuse, I got involved in a very performance-based religion. I learned that even though,

'Jesus had paid it all' he left some debt to me. I had to be a good girl to maintain my good standing with God.

That only further cemented the idea that I had to perform. And by God, perform I did.

I became an overachiever, a really hard worker; I was there early, ready to go, ready to please, ready to earn my keep.

When my husband was wandering around in the first seven years of our marriage, unsure of who he wanted to be when he grew up, I worked enough to cover both of us financially.

I proved to the world that I was worth being here. I worked for it. I earned it and so, I was worthwhile.

When I got sick and I couldn't work as much, and those few family members judged me so terribly, I got the opportunity to ask myself if they were right, '*Am* I more worth loving when I work hard and provide? *Is* my worth tied to my productivity?'

Oh god, it was hard. But it was valuable. I needed to come to the conclusion that my value was inherent just in being here. That I had my own shit to deal with and grow in. I realized that my friends and family were just projecting their unhappiness and judgment in my direction.

I finally didn't need to be a victim to them anymore, because I stopped being a victim to me. Their unkindness was an important part of my journey because it was my opportunity to know my own value. I needed to sort that out so that I didn't fall prey to anyone else's opinion of me. When you hold your own high opinion of yourself and know your inestimable value, you're not a victim – not to yourself or to anyone else.

And you're not even a victim to your diagnosis.

2. You get the opportunity to see your reflection.

There's this idea that everyone in our life is a reflection of the beliefs we hold about ourselves. That the external playground of people in your sandbox is simply a reflection of your own self-beliefs.

I had the opportunity to examine whether or not these folks, who were being harsh and rejecting of me, were merely external representations of an inner voice that was part of my inner story.

I'm not sure if all of that is true. But I will tell you, it has been valuable for me to consider because, honestly, it takes my eyes off of them as a person, and it puts the attention on the bigger issue: to heal and address that voice of condemnation that still lives within me.

So, when one of the family members was being nasty or unkind about me regarding health stuff, I had the opportunity to look and see where *I* was being nasty and unkind to me. If that person was just playing out loud the tape of negativity that was already in my head, then, I didn't really need to address that person as my first order of business. I needed to address me first.

You're Not Crazy and You're Not Alone

What did I say about myself in my private thoughts?

Oh man, it was not kind.

It was about how fat, ugly or unproductive I was. About how I wasn't strong enough to get out of this health spiral. It was about how I was failing my husband, kids, and God.

It was one sentence after another, screwing with my mind, all. day. long.

One of my favorite big thinkers is author Byron Katie. She said in her book, Loving What Is: "I don't have to let go of any negative thoughts anymore, I simply greet them with understanding and they let go of me."

I came to a point where instead of doing my old religious thinking of trying to resist that "evil" thought, instead I greeted it with understanding.

I said to myself, 'Stacey, of course you think that way and you demand a lot of yourself. You were such a great student of life and your teachers taught that you had to work for your worth.'

You had to redefine truth, as you knew it, so that you could still be loved by the people who didn't want to hear your truth. Those people taught you that loyalty to them meant surrender of yourself. You had to give up being you, in order to be loved.

You had to keep quiet about the abuses that were happening so that you wouldn't be rejected. You were taught that really well, and you were a good student of that.

With a Family Member Like That, Who Needs an Enemy

If you had been taught something different, you would have learned that. But you learned this instead. You don't need that old thinking anymore, it doesn't serve you anymore because you're aware of this: when you know who you are, no one can take that away from you. So, you don't have to perform any-more. You don't have to worry about risking their love because now, you are loving yourself ...'

And those thoughts would bring a *sigh* to me. I'd exhale the old belief as quickly as a breath. There was nothing to resist because the presence of Love and Understanding released the negativity.

It was an ongoing process, and still is in some ways. There are still buttons that get pushed, but overall, greeting those nega-tive thoughts with understanding helps me to be free of them. And since it was the unkindness of the people closest to me who were reflecting that voice, my practice of seeing them as a mirror ended up serving me in my healing.

Please know that what you just read right there, has taken me quite some time to work through. Some bits came in an in-stant, but much of it unfolded over a longer stretch. Be patient with yourself. Greet yourself and your reflection with under-standing.

3. You get the opportunity to grow in your Divine humanity.

The truth is that we all screw up. We all judge. We all presume and misunderstand and reject. We just do. It's part of the hu-man experience. You're a card-carrying member. Welcome.

You're Not Crazy and You're Not Alone

And when I got sick and went on a spiritual journey to look at my belief systems about life, love and God, I got some epiphanies that changed my life.

One of them was:

God is Love. And Love made me. Therefore I AM Love.

That's it.

There was nothing more I needed to work for, or do, or perform.

I got clear that the Divine and I were intertwined and you could no more take the fact that I'm a female out of my being than you could take the Divine out of my essence.

Yes, there are events and messages that can either support our inherent value or interrupt our belief in that. Like the sexual abuse, it affected how I saw myself as a woman, but it didn't change the fact that I am female.

In the same way, we can have life events and messages interrupt the idea that we are of the Divine, but that doesn't mean that God is any less within us.

Once I got clear on the Love message, the old religious 'them and us' bullshit went away. I didn't need to save people or change them. They weren't broken, so I didn't need to fix them. Being sick and going through that spiritual questioning about 'Who Am I?' And coming to the conclusion that 'I Am Love' didn't just transform me, it transformed how I saw my connection to other people.

The family members who were being rude to me? We're all threaded together by the same Source of Love and Mystery. If they knew how amazing they were and that they didn't have to perform for love, they would live that out with others, including me.

My youngest son asked me one day, "Mom, how come you invite that person over even when sometimes they're not very kind to you?"

I said, "Well, first of all, I love that person and I know that they love me. They have other things going on in their life that make them cranky. I feel strong enough right now, to be around them and to love them."

"And second of all, I want you to know that I'm okay to invite them over or to not invite them over. I'm peaceful either way. If someone is being dangerous or unnecessarily hurtful, I don't want them around. Trust me.

And if I have invited them over and they start being rude or mean, I address it or I just walk away. It's okay to speak up for yourself and it's okay love someone and still walk away when they're not treating you right. The connection is in here..." I pointed to my heart, "but that doesn't mean we always know how to be connected in our relationships."

I made sure I said it a couple of ways to him, because that walking away part has been a big lesson for me.

Because you can't truly welcome someone into your heart and life until you're crystal clear that you are able to walk away when it's toxic. That's what freedom is and true Love is about freedom. Understanding we are all threaded together is vital to our compassion and perspective, yes. Because that allows you to walk away from someone with the grace that says, "It's not time, and we're not ready…" Instead of walking away with, "I'm right and they're the big honkin' asshole and always will be."

Being committed to me, and loving myself means that I know when to stay and I know when to leave. Loving myself is the foundation for loving every. other. person in my life.

It's a lesson I'm still learning but I can say this, I'm grateful to be able to see that we're all connected to the Light and Love that created us, even if we haven't figured how to live in that reality, and can't see it in ourselves…

Yet.

4. You get the opportunity to represent your own voice.

For many years I was quiet when someone would treat me poorly. Then, I would want my husband to stand up for me. He wasn't great at that. He had people-pleasing issues. That pushed my buttons of unworthiness.

One day, the question came to me in meditation, "Why are you waiting for him to protect you and represent you when you're not even willing to protect and represent yourself? Why are you expecting him to see your worth when you don't even know your own?"

Again, sheesh, life is really our opportunity to grow.

I wanted my husband to stand up for me – he was my *family*.

The gift in him not standing up for me was my opportunity to look at where my belief came from. A lot was from my unworthiness, but also from my religious experience that told me that the man had to be John Wayne morning, noon, and night and I had to be some damsel in distress.

When I was younger, I was told by my abuser, a drug dealer in town, that I had to keep what happened a secret.

I was told by my parents, that I couldn't share about the tensions going on inside the home.

I was told by the church, that I couldn't stand up for myself.

I was such a good student. I really was. And I was a victim to my own beliefs about myself and therefore I was in relationships where I remained the victim. I learned to not truly stand up for myself. Oh, I knew how to be sarcastic and I knew how to take things out on me by being hard on myself. I knew how to over-control parts of my life so that I wouldn't feel so out of control. But all of those things, in my understanding, were part of an overcompensating way of dealing with the fact that I wasn't representing my own voice.

Because I didn't know my own value.

You're Not Crazy and You're Not Alone

Because I didn't realize the Divine in me.

I don't have to defend myself anymore. Oh, I'm learning to represent myself, but that's different than living in a chronically defensive mode. Chronic defense comes from a belief that you're always the victim and someone else is always the perpetrator. Being defensive is a posture that is reactive to an attack.

I don't need to prove to anyone that I'm sick – and god, who even wants to take the role of the lawyer trying to prove how sick you are? Because you know what happens when you take that role? You get sicker just to prove that you're really sick.

We are powerful people.

One day, it dawned on me that perhaps my thyroid was waving the little white flag to get attention. That it was trying to say something.

Something that I wasn't willing to say with my voice.

And I wondered if all those years of not speaking my peace, made my thyroid anxious and sick.

And if not using my voice, made my thyroid 'speak up' instead.

I started realizing that I used my sickness to be my voice because I didn't feel comfortable putting my feelings, wants, and needs out there. I felt vulnerable to say, "I feel angry." Or "I don't want to go to that party and hang out with those people." Or "I need to take some time for myself."

With a Family Member Like That, Who Needs an Enemy

I was afraid of being questioned, disregarded, or rejected.

So, instead of being angry, my thyroid would go into a 'flare' and start sticking out of my neck.

Instead of saying "No" to the party, I would end up sick and would have to decline.

Instead of saying I needed time, I would find myself incredibly exhausted from the Hashimoto's and would end up in bed. Alone.

I'm not saying all of those symptoms weren't real. I just started wondering if any of my sickness was rooted in – or exacerbated by – me not using my voice.

I'd begin to softly stroke my thyroid in a comforting and grateful way and say, "Thank you for waving the white flag. Thanks for letting me know that I need to take care of some business about loving myself. Thank you for helping me to see that I need to not only be conscious of what I put into my mouth, but what comes out of it, as well.
I am committing to using my voice to say what I want, what I need, and what I feel so that you don't have to take on more than you need to."

I started saying what I felt.
I started stating what I wanted.
I started asking for what I needed.

I will tell you that a completely different energy came to me. It takes a lot of energy to hold back your own voice. All that energy I had repressed was starting to come up in a good way. I felt very alive.

Self-expression is life-giving.

So, regarding the family stuff and the practice of using your voice? Just be aware:

Everyone is not necessarily going to understand. It's just life.

Know yourself – that you are of the Divine, that you are dealing with an autoimmune thing, and that you are of great value.

Represent, not defend, yourself, and speak your peace.

If someone can't be at peace with you, you take your peace and walk away. No one has a right to take your peace.

Unless you give it to them.

Don't give it to them.

Speak your peace.

5. You get the opportunity to forgive

I think the sentence from number four fits for this one, too: everyone screws up. We all hurt each other. The human existence includes some pain.

Forgiveness, in my mind, is not something you give when you

feel like it; it's something you choose when it's needed.

Now, I'm not suggesting we ignore our feelings of hurt or anger or any of that. I'm just suggesting we honor the feeling without reacting to it. We have our feeling and want to respond in a way that is alignment with our integrity. Lashing out at someone who's being an asshole isn't going to make you feel better (well, at least not long-term) about it. You know you. Maybe you're prone to guilt.

Be angry. Be hurt. Give that emotion a place that's safe to be.

I'm just saying in the middle of that completely shitty feeling, choose forgiveness.

For example: I have stood in front of the mirror or sat in the car and said, "I choose to forgive that person. I don't want to. I'm pissed. They hurt me and they were being a complete asshole/Orange Cone/whatever. I just choose to. The feelings will come later."

And then, this deep sigh of the high vibration of truth happens in my body.

Now, some people would say, "Oh, you should only forgive when you're ready." I get that. I so get that whole idea of feeling your feeling. But I also know that for me, sometimes my feelings lead me to something grand and sometimes, my feelings hook up with my OCD, fixated thinking and I spiral down. So, knowing me and what serves me best, in the middle of my feelings, I have to make a *conscious* choice.

You're Not Crazy and You're Not Alone

Like just the other day, I was in the shower and these thoughts started messing with my head. Thoughts of this person who hurt me and then, that person who jumped on that bandwagon of judgment. It was old shit. Something stirred my pot and this is what came to the surface. It wouldn't have served me to go down that road. I recognized that the thought was more of a habit and a distraction than anything else. So, I just closed my eyes under the running water and said, "I forgive them. I bless them. I choose to release myself from that negativity. I send blessings their way and my way."

Now that was in the middle of a memory – these were old hurts, resurfacing and not new hurts happening. Choosing to forgive, bless, and release stops the maddening cycle in my brain.

But in the middle of an injury – when the heart and trust are broken and the person on the other end hasn't stopped the hurtful behavior – we all know how unbelievably emotionally messy that can be.

I reach a point in the middle of my strong feelings where I recognize that a choice would be a powerful thing to make and I will speak out load, to no one but me, "I choose to forgive. I don't feel like that now. But I'm willing for this to be a forgiven and healed situation." Then, the space of willingness is open and I am expressing my commitment to be in a state of forgiveness. Sort of like Babe Ruth, pointing to the far bleachers over the outfield. He put his intention out there before he ever addressed the ball. Putting an intention of forgiveness is pointing and aiming to the healing in your future.

With a Family Member Like That, Who Needs an Enemy

Plus, being in that state of willingness, allows me to breathe and heal. I may have feelings of being trapped, but I'm declaring to my self and the Universe, that I am not willing to be trapped by unforgiveness. That will help me to walk in freedom.

At some point, the feelings of relief will follow.

I still allow myself to be angry -- which is REALLY hard for me. I must have made some kind of altar in my life to 'Not Being Angry' so, it's super uncomfortable for me to feel pissed. And man, it's hard to be emotionally potty-trained on some of this stuff when you're in your thirties and forties – when you've got all this baggage tied to not being angry.

Sometimes you overshoot it by overdoing the anger thing, and then you have to apologize to the other person, even though they were the one who acted like a weenie in the first place. Or you feel guilty for feeling angry and then, you have to apologize to yourself for not allowing yourself to be mad.

It's all kinds of fun.

Sigh.

And, in related news: I still allow myself to be *sad* which is another emotion that is tricky for me. I was told I was over-sensitive so much in my life. I tried to change but didn't know how. During the overwhelming abuse, I ended up cutting off my connection to my heart. Sad seemed to go away. I didn't feel anything.

You're Not Crazy and You're Not Alone

Because instead of sad and oversensitive, I chose 'numb.'

Numb will get you through a season, but learning how to feel the full range of emotions, including sadness, helps you grow as a human being.

So in the space of those feelings, sad and angry, I choose to forgive.

One of my favorite quotes came from a Vanity Fair interview with Monica Lewinksy. Monica, in my mind was, forever and only, going to be associated with a stained dress, a big cigar and the Oval Office ...until I read this interview.

In it, she was asked two questions that stood out to me:

"What is the greatest gift you've ever received?"

Her answer was, "Forgiveness."

"What is the greatest gift you've ever given?"

Her answer was, "My heart."

I believe they're both connected. When we finally allow ourselves to be connected to our heart and honor that, we are able to be safe enough to extend one of the greatest gifts we could ever give to someone else: *forgiveness.*

When we forgive that family member who has hurt us by their misunderstanding or misjudgment, we are giving them a gift, yes – but we are finally giving ourselves the gifts of

Connection to our own heart,

And healing,

And moving on.

6. You get the opportunity to be gracious

I believe in 'going long' with people. It's a term that I remember from when my dad and I would either play football together or we'd watch our favorite New York Giants play their games.

Instead of short passes to gain distance on the field, sometimes the quarterback would hold onto the ball and the receiver would 'go long.'

The receiver would run as far and deep as the play dictated and then, this gorgeous pass would soar above everyone's heads and land in the pocket of his arm. The long pass was a risk – because the extra time it took for both the quarterback and the receiver to get in position left a lot of room for a hard tackle and a missed play – but it allowed maximum opportunity for an epic touchdown.

With my family, I definitely see the value of little passes ...making daily investments, little by little, over time. But in this analogy, I'm talking about overlooking some of those offenses that could snag you and wear you down, little-by-little, and instead of addressing every single thing, opting to 'go long.'

It's about thinking of the long term relationship and trusting that over time, what they can't see right now in me, my good character and my deep love, eventually will be seen by them as life unfolds.

The value in that for me is this: I don't want to get into performance mode with anyone in my family so that they'll love me more. Trying to course-correct for every little thing they think about me, or feel about me, is going to wear me out and it's NOT my vision for how I want to live life. I don't want to react to every false accusation. I don't want to address every small thing. That's small thinking. I have a bigger vision for my life AND for the relationship.

But the other great thing is this: it gives me an opportunity to keep my eye on my long-term goal and it allows me the opportunity to be gracious.

One day, they may end up with a diagnosis the same or similar as mine. I don't ever wish that upon anyone. But if it did happen, I would be honored to be the one they come to so that I could support and love them in the process. Even though they didn't have the compassion to do that for me, I have to live in the enlightenment I have. And I would be grateful to be trusted with someone's heart on this journey of healing if they ever needed that help.

And honestly, that did happen. A family member who had been judging of me did call with this diagnosis. And it was my honor to love and support them through it. I had no glee in their distress. I ached for them because I knew what it felt like. I always said, "If what I'm learning the long way could, in turn, help someone I love dearly, it would be so worth it."

With a Family Member Like That, Who Needs an Enemy

I shortcut them as best I knew how. And what knowledge I had accrued had served them so well that they were on the road to recovery in a matter of a months.

I won't always be this sick or feel this broken or be this misunderstood. I am going long with myself and with the people in my life.

So here's the deal:

Family is its own mixed bag of tricks: it's wonderful, committed and crazy when it's at its best. And when it's hurtful and at its worst, it's an opportunity.

The family you're born with is an important part of your life, love and spiritual journey.

And please remember this: when your own family and you are in a crappy space, there is other "family" that appears in unexpected places.

- That friend who will come and sit with you – again – when the remedies don't work.
- That neighbor who will make you a cup of tea.
- That stranger who shares health tips with you at the Farmer's Market.
- And now, the collage of Facebook friends and Hashimoto's groups, like Hashimoto's 411, that are here for each other.

You're Not Crazy and You're Not Alone

All of these people have very family-like qualities.

If your family isn't really there for you, don't focus on that, or on them. When you think of them, just bless them, forgive them and learn from them.

Look for where 'family-like' love and care *is* appearing and express gratitude for that.

Please hear me, on behalf of all of us with an autoimmune disease, especially if you are a family member who has helped and were kind and were gracious along the way: your gifts of kindness and support were beautiful and amazing.

Not everyone, though, was like you. You stood out in a crowd.

And so did they.

I, personally, have learned grace and generosity and kindness from you. And I have learned healing, self-representation, and forgiveness because of the others.

Thank you for your love in the process.

And for those who weren't kind, thank you for the reminder that you need love, too.

And for reminding me that always, no matter what,
I need to love myself.

Chapter 12

Fear, Fi, Fo, Fum...

You know, I'm an Italian. From New Jersey. Who was raised Catholic.

We're crazy.
We're passionate.
And we love to eat.

We pretty much consumed four things in life:

Pasta
Bread
Cheese
And
Fear

Yup. Fear.

Mass consumption of scary stories told by the old Italian ladies, sitting around the kitchen table, drinking black demitasse and crunching on homemade anisette biscotti.

They'd dunk a little cookie, tell a little horror story about Vincenzo who fell from the roof after he saw a black cat. About Maurizio who got bit by a spider and died after he got in a fight with his mother. And about Cugentina who sister's husband's brother died after she counted all the cars in a funeral procession.

And then, everyone would say, "God forbid!" and make the sign of the cross over themselves.

You think I'm kidding...

We had superstitions that I had never heard of before. My grandmother was terrified of birds. "Birds bring bad news, Stacey!" She'd say in her New Jersey accent, taking a long draw on her mentholated cigarette. "But black birds," she paused and took another drag, "they bring news of *death*." She whispered the last word like the birds were going to hear and come flocking like a scene from the infamous Alfred Hitchcock movie.

One day, she saw a crow on the back patio. Oh my Lord. She ran in, turned off the lights, closed the drapes and pushed me into the pantry to hide with her. The phone started ringing on the wall in the kitchen so, I moved to answer it, "No! Don't answer the phone."

I looked at her and wondered if she thought the birds were calling. I also wondered if we were going to have to live in the pantry forever.

My family was a hoot. They were intensely committed to their food, their faith and their fears. They were big-time experts on how to scare each other half to death in a single bound.

Like when I was getting ready to be knocked out to get my wisdom teeth pulled when I was 17. One of my family members was talking to another one, right in front of me,

Fear-Fi-Fo-Fum...

"Oh my god! Remember the story about the little boy who went to the dentist to have his tooth pulled out and instead of putting the Novocaine in the syringe for his mouth, they put it in the IV bag where the anesthesia was supposed to be! He died right there! It froze his heart! God forbid!"

Then, they made the sign of the cross.

Meanwhile, I'm sitting there about to go in to have a needle shoved in my arm and I'm sweating and praying it's not the last time that I see these crazy people. Alive.

Yeah.

Fear was our food.

And we were fed a feast daily.

Fear and Faith

So, it made perfect sense when I started exploring other religions to add to my Catholic experience (which I loved by the way, and no, I'm not kidding), I ended up finding a religion that was very fear-based. It was focused VERY MUCH on a God who loved me, as long I did things the right way. But if not, BAM! Injury, death or worse, dis-ease. All of my imperfections and sinful disobedience, building up to the crescendo of going to hell, forever and ever, amen.

This God who was supposed to love me seemed very easy to piss off. And he held quite a grudge.

You're Not Crazy and You're Not Alone

For sort of like…forever.

That brought a lot of fear. Because it's one thing to not want to step on a crack to break your mother's back. It's a whole other thing to not want to step out of line with God and end up bursting into flames.

Fear and Health Issues

So, you add my superstitious upbringing with my superstitious faith and then, throw in an undiagnosed thyroid issue that had a long run of misdiagnoses, sitting in doctors offices, having scary tests, having terrifying symptoms like heart arrhythmias and a host of other weird things you can't easily figure out, and basically you can understand why…

I was scared half to death.

I felt so chronically guilty and on the verge of hell. And now, I was sick. No doctor could figure me out.

I looked for so many answers. At hospitals, clinics, self-help centers, therapy, churches, mind/body/spirit places …

And because I hadn't come to a place of inner peace in my life, the whole process of this health journey was a fear-fest. I got on planes I was afraid to fly on, to go to places I was afraid to be at, to learn from people I was afraid were going to tell me something horrible about 'me, my health and I' …

I was afraid of, yet again, being told it was anxiety and I was afraid of being told it was something worse.

I was afraid of knowing and afraid of not-knowing.

That was compounded by the family folks who were being rejecting because I wasn't 'me' anymore and a husband who honestly didn't get it. Oh, he loved me, but he was in his own world with his own problems.

Alone was a terrible place to be.

Alone with me.
Alone with these symptoms.
Alone with my morbid imagination.
Alone with a scary-ass god.

I slept night after night, in my car, in the parking lot of the emergency room at the local hospital. That's how bad it was.

I didn't want to die alone, next to my husband who was checked out of reality.

I didn't want to die with a rude family member who only loved me when I made more money and didn't inconvenience them.

I didn't want to die with my religious friends around me who were always trying to figure out what sin I had committed (oh, and I was just like them, trust me.)

None of those things comforted me.

So, I slept walking distance from the ER for months, so that at

You're Not Crazy and You're Not Alone

least someone who was *required* to take care of me, would.

I just wanted some comfort.

I wanted someone I could trust.

I wanted someone who would validate that what was going on inside of my body was just not right.

I wanted someone to say, "You don't have to live a perfect life with a perfect heart in order to be a healthy person. You're allowed to make mistakes and be a growing person."

I wanted someone to say to me,

"You're not crazy.

and you're not alone...

And I will help."

I'm sitting here with tears in my eyes as I write this. I've avoided this chapter until the very end and almost considered leaving it out. Because it's hard to go back there. In order to write from the heart, you have to go back into the center of the situation you're telling about in order to feel it authentically.

I had to go back into that dark space of the fear and anxiety to write this chapter. I was not looking forward to it.

But if you don't feel it authentically, you don't write it authentically and then, no one gets that you *get* it.

Fear-Fi-Fo-Fum...

No one feels understood.

So, through bleary-teary eyes I want to tell you: I get it.

The alone-ness and Fear feels enormous, relentless and end-less.

You wonder if you're ever going to feel good again.

You wonder if your health is going to be there for you in your old age. Or even next year.

Or even tomorrow.

You wonder if you're just the biggest selfish ass in the world for wanting your husband to understand and be more of your ad-vocate. Or you wonder if he's the biggest ass for needing to be begged to pay attention to you. To help you. To research with you. To be compassionate to you.

You wonder if you're worth being loved.
Worth being healthy.
Worth being healed.

You wonder if this is some cosmic burp that blew in your direction or if you really screwed up big time and you're being punished.

You wonder if you're going to ever get to have kids or if you do, you wonder if your kids will get this autoimmune thing. That would be horrible and you know you wouldn't wish Hashimoto's on anyone ...

… okay, maybe just a few of the people who were assholes to you about this whole health thing, but then you think about it and you realize, *No …not even them. I wouldn't even wish this on them.*

You do a lot of wondering.

And a lot of overthinking.

Because you're afraid.

I want to tell you this:

You're not alone.

Valuable Questions to Help You Down Off the Ledge of Insanity

Hashimoto's can come with a host of symptoms, including the ever-so-delightful one of anxiety. *Sigh.* Here are some things that you can do when you're feeling anxious and outside of yourself.

The first thing I do is grab a glass of water, step outside if I can, and ask myself some questions.

Is my thyroid off?

The swinging nature of Hashimoto's can throw you into a hyper flare or a hypo state. That can give you palpitations and make you sweat and feel like you're going crazy. Here's the deal: it takes time for the meds to adjust. Get in touch with your health professional to see what can help you in the meantime of the adjustment.

Fear-Fi-Fo-Fum...

Am I hydrated?

One of the main symptoms of under-hydration is anxiety. Drink a glass or two of pure water.

Am I having a food reaction?

Do you know that one of the side effects of food sensitivity is palpitations and anxiety?

Am I tired?

Not getting enough quality sleep is an anxiety stimulant.

Are my hormones changing?

The flux in hormones can affect the homeostasis of our peace.

And I keep going with other questions:

Am I not expressing myself?

When I don't speak my peace, it becomes my anxiety. It's important to be true to our voice. The lie is you have to say it perfectly. You don't. You also don't have to be a wretched ass about it, but once you allow yourself the permission to self-express, you will say things in a way that aligns with you. That, alone, can calm you. Speak your truth.

You're Not Crazy and You're Not Alone

Am I feeling the energy of other people or life events going on?

One of the other ones that's kind of woo-woo but I'm gonna say it anyway because you already know I kinda am ...sometimes I can get anxious just being around the energy of other people. I'm a sensitive person and for me to go to Disneyland or the grocery store, or a movie theater, or whatever can be the most overstimulating experience for my senses.

Plus, I'm an intuitive person. That's part of what makes me a really good coach to people. I can feel what they're feeling and put it into words that give it life and bring freedom as we explore. But when I am in that sensitive state, I can feel the energy of other people, or even of events in the world. Just ask my husband how many times I turn to him right before an earthquake and say, "We're about to have an earthquake." He'll tell you.

So sometimes, my anxiety isn't even coming from me.

Am I in a relationship that is out of balance?

Just acknowledging a toxic or out-of-balance relationship can help to bring an inner peace. Sometimes the anxiety is coming simply from hiding the truth from ourselves.

Be honest about where your relationships are at. Even if you choose to stay in some crazy ones for a while, you'll at least be free of the lie that it's a healthy relationship when it's really not. The next steps will unfold. Self-honestly is a peaceful and self-honoring first step.

Fear-Fi-Fo-Fum...

Am I doing a protocol for my health that is out of alignment with my beliefs?

Sometimes we choose to do things that do not seem right, but we feel technically disqualified from questioning it or addressing our concerns with the health professional. When we allow our intuition to come back into our world, we learn how to honor that inner voice that says, "This doesn't feel good." When we humbly bring that out on the table we are able to represent and honor that voice within us. When that happens, it gets stronger. When that happens, WE get stronger.

Practice using your voice. It is health to you.

Am I having a belief about the process of life, or my faith in God, that is rooted in a fearful place?

When you address the core of your beliefs, you get to see that which is coming from Love and that which is coming from Fear.

Being able to track back to our foundation helps us to see what beliefs we've built our lives upon. This is not for the faint of heart, because our whole life can end up getting get uprooted by the discovery that we have been living on a foundation made of Fear. Recognize those Fear-based formulas, they look like this: "If you act this way, look this way, talk this way, perform this way, pray this way ...THEN, you'll be loved. But if you don't. Then, you won't."

It takes a hunger for freedom to look at this with honesty.

Am I holding unforgiveness toward someone, including my-self?

To hold on to a grudge can be a huge source of anxiety. We are feeling the energy of another person's life hermetically sealed to ours. Forgiveness is like that Goo-Gone stuff – it just removes those stuck things in our life. Like people who were being wee-nies.

Or to ourselves when the weenie hat is on us.

You know, when you're giving yourself a relentlessly hard time. When all you can see about yourself is what you've done wrong and you're not letting yourself off the hook for anything. Yeah. That creates anxiety.

I sometimes find myself saying, "I choose to forgive me. Not just for what I did, but for expecting myself to be perfect in all things. That's a heavy load and I release myself from that burden."

That's not an exhaustive list but it's a pretty good one.

A Quick Word On Panic Attacks

A dear friend of mine and her husband just visited for the week-end, Marriage Family Therapist, Carol Meadors. She and I were talking about this chapter in the book. She said, "Oh, I always tell my clients, if they're having a panic attack to invite more of the fear they're feeling into their space."

I started laughing, thinking she was joking. I looked over. She wasn't.

"Oh yeah, Stacey, you think I'm kidding? I'm not! See, a panic attack has you feeling completely out of control – sweaty, heart racing, feeling like you're going to jump out of your skin and it's never going to end." I nodded. Been there. Done that. Bought the t-shirt. Wanted to strangle myself with it.

"Well, when you're feeling that out of control and then, you invite more of that experience in, you're actually taking control. When that happens, the panic vanishes."

So, tuck that little tip into your toolbox for the next time you feel like you're on the ledge, okay?

And send me an e-mail about how it worked for you.

No, really, I'm serious.

All that to say, fear (the deep-rooted issues that need to heal) and anxiety (the situational issues that need to change) are not fun at all, but they can be part of the ride for many of us with Hashimoto's.

I want you to know that there is an end to this Fear/Anxiety tunnel you feel you're in. It's not always going to be like this. There are practical things you can do like I mentioned above and in other chapters:

You're Not Crazy and You're Not Alone

- Step outside to put your feet in the earth.
- Drink some water.
- Eat foods on your program.
- Do deep breathing.
- Do the Jin Shin Jyutsu finger holds, meditate, or pray.
- Express yourself in an honest, clear, and honoring way.
- Check on your meds and supplements to see that something isn't jacking you up.

And yeah, do the inner work to look at where stuff comes from. Take that journey to getting to the lie that's living in the Fear – and find your way to the truth that's in Love.

When my boys were little, I used to ask them what the opposite of Up was, they'd say, "Down" and the opposite of High, they'd say, "Low." And the opposite of Love, and they'd say, "Not Love."

Fear
is 'Not Love.'

If anything is holding you hostage and convincing you to believe that you are not worth this life here on earth. I want you to know, that's a lie.

That lie is 'Not Love' and it is coming from Fear.

Ask the Divine in you, that valuable question, 'Show me who I am. Help me to see myself the way you see me?' And watch the most amazing journey unfold.

Fear-Fi-Fo-Fum...

Truth lives in Love.
And Love wants you free.

Love knows how to get you there.

Seek Love.

Chapter 13

The Landmines of Mercury and Iodine (Hey! That Kinda Rhymes...)

Okay, so here's the deal. If you're new to this whole Hashimoto's thing, let me be the first to tell you: removing mercury fillings and taking iodine when you have Hashimoto's are two controversial subjects.

For those long-timers with Hashimoto's, you already know what I'm talking about.

I have done both. Had some fillings removed (due to the possible mercury toxicity concerns in the old amalgams.)

And I've taken iodine while having Hashimoto's.

While I have had my experiences AND I have my opinions, I do NOT believe this is a one-size-fits-all kind of decision. I could persuade you with my personal stories on both of these issues, but that is not my heart in this at all. I desire to expose you to information that may not be coming along the traditional paths, and then, empower you to make the best decisions for *you*.

Because this book sheds light on the emotional issues that affect us, here is all I basically want to say about this to encourage you and support you emotionally through this process:

Don't jump on a bandwagon. There are the 'always do this' and 'never do that' groups in both camps.

Please, please, please – just seek wisdom, do research and do what is best for YOU, even if your best girlfriend has Hashimoto's and goes down one path, reserve your right to listen to what's Wisdom and Peace to you.

When you hear a doctor hold to one thought and not the other, just check out the other side's thought.

Fear can drive us to do things that Wisdom wouldn't lead us to do.

Seek wisdom.

I'm listing, below, some resources that I trust.

Iodine:

Interview with Dr. Eric Osansky and Dr. David Brownstein: http://www.naturalendocrinesolutions.com/archives/an-interview-with-dr-david-brownstein-on-iodine-and-thyroid-health

The Landmines of Mercury and Iodine

Dr. Datis Kharrazian:
http://thyroidbook.com/blog/iodine-and-hashimotos

Truth Calkins:
https://www.facebook.com/ThyroidHealth

Sharon Tenpenny:
http://tenpennyimc.com/thyroid-conditions/hashimotos-thy-roiditis

Chris Kresser:
http://chriskresser.com/iodine-for-hypothyroidism-like-gaso-line-on-a-fire

Mercury:

What is Mercury: http://www.deq.state.ok.us/factsheets/land/whatismercury.pdf

Dr. Hal Huggins: http://www.hugginsappliedhealing.com

Andrew Cutler PhD PE: http://www.noamalgam.com

All is well.

With all things, my desire is to listen to the Wisdom that resounds for me in this season (recognizing that Wisdom might change in the next) and to walk in that. If something doesn't resound, I do what is peace to me.

You're Not Crazy and You're Not Alone

And I want to highly encourage you and empower you to do the same:

Listen for Wisdom

And you will find Peace.

Follow Peace.

Chapter 14

Wisdoms That Saved My Bacon

You know how some great wisdom finds you and you're like, 'Yeah! I want to write that down so I remember!' Well, this is that little chapter that has a few worth noting.

1. Hiatal Valve.

> I really can't tell you enough how invaluable this bit of information has been to me. I will forever be thankful to my dear, long-time friend and brilliant Chiropractor Dr. Ralph Umbriaco for teaching me about this.
>
> I had symptoms of palpitations, nausea, GERD, pain in my chest, pain down my arm and fogginess in my head. As you know, I went to the ER several times, and the cardiologist, AND had the stress test and more tests than I, or my insurance company could count.
>
> I finally went to see Ralph. He did his energy work (NAET) magic and said, "Your toxicity is high. You must be feeling like poop." He's so real in the middle of all that brilliance. He tested some more, "And your valve is open."

You're Not Crazy and You're Not Alone

No clue what that meant.

He explained that the hiatal valve is the great mimicker. You can feel like you're having a heart attack, gall bladder attack, anxiety, difficulty breathing and a host of other symptoms, all when your valve is open.

He laid me down on the table and told me to turn my head. Then, he proceeded to close my valve, which is not too far from the sternum and requires pushing down and pulling down in a way that made me want to kick him between the legs. Didn't feel good. He did it three times. Hurt more every time. I sat up. Palpitations gone, pain in chest and arm gone. Nausea gone. Had a little bruise in my belly but I felt like a scrillion bucks.

Now, you read about how I used to sleep in the hospital parking lot, right? It was for these same symptoms. I can't tell you how many times I went to the ER thinking I was having a heart attack (I wasn't) when it was probably something as simply remedied as an open valve.

I looked at Ralph and said, "Do you know how many times I've been to the ER for feeling *this* lousy and no one *ever* mentioned an open valve? How come?"

He nodded in his good-natured way, "Valve issues are super common, Stacey but the overwhelming majority of doctors don't have a clue as to how to identify them or treat them."

I felt so grateful to know this wisdom about the hiatal valve, as Ralph showed my husband and me how to close my own valve when the symptoms got triggered in the future. All the best doctors in my life, like Ralph Umbriaco, empower their patients to do as much as they can on their own.

I really honor that.

I also feel sad for how many folks are running around feeling terrible and it's something as simply treated as an open valve. We gotta spread the word. I'm going to tell Ralph to do a You-Tube video for all of us, okay?

And of course I have to put the disclaimer here: if you're having scary-ass symptoms, I am NOT telling you to NOT go to the hospital or NOT call your doctor. I am telling you MY story of what wisdom I found after I had exhausted all those other avenues and no one had an answer for me.

Which leads me to another wisdom that Ralph taught me:

2. Think Horses Not Zebras

I can't tell you how many times I thought I had Zambu Fever or something scary and exotic, especially after looking up my symptoms on the Internet. Looking stuff up on the Internet is a mixed bag of tricks: sometimes you find the answer you need and it encourages you, but most of the time, not so much. You look up "How to Remove A Splinter" and suddenly you read that you're dying. On the World Wide Web, all roads seem to lead to death...

And pornography.

You're Not Crazy and You're Not Alone

But, mostly death.
Not very helpful.

So, Dr. Umbriaco's tip was very helpful to my anxious, over-thinking mind when I was feeling 23,000 aches and pains, ALL related to the undiagnosed Hashimoto's, and *all* in the middle of the night with no one there to help me. When you're having a symptom, don't think of something exotic that lives in Africa like a zebra, think of something simpler that is local, like a horse.

Think:
- Is my valve open?
- Am I under-hydrated?
- What did I last eat?
- When did I last eat?

And do something like have a cup of tea or step outside for some fresh air, or do something to distract you.

Not that I'm a fan of distraction but, it will prove a point to you: if you can turn on The Food Network to be distracted and your symptoms go away, the symptoms were coming from your mind and not Zambu Fever.

So here's the deal: thinking that you have the worst possible thing isn't going to help you have sweet dreams. If anxiety is making you think the symptom is the worst thing possible, take on the idea that whatever is wrong is something simple and easily remedied. In that space of peace, you will be more able to hear wisdom about what to do.

Wisdoms that Saved My Bacon

3. Jin Shin Jyutsu

It sounds like a martial art but it's not. It's a Japanese modality of healing, that my dear friend, Joni August, introduced to me several years ago. She has used it for decades, practices it daily with great results, and has studied it with people from all over the world. I had never heard of it before and I have to say, it has been such a tremendous gift to my life.

Jin Shin is what some describe as 'energy work'. The basic premise is that there is a blueprint for your optimal health or 'flow' where you are functioning at your strongest - and then, there's the reality of the state your body is in – which is not always so flow-y.

Different things affect our energetic flow: our emotions, our body's injuries and sicknesses, our relationships, and our perceptions about life to name a few.

By using your hands as your own 'jumper cables', Jin Shin instructs that you can help the places that are 'stuck' and therefore help with pain, sickness and dis-ease. The work is to line you up with that optimal blueprint by placing your hands at strategic parts of your body with certain 'holds' to help restore your mind/body/spirit flow. I'll give you an example of how this helped me:

One day in the middle of trying to put on a four-day charity event, homeschooling my children, and working two at-home businesses, I went to make my bed. I should have jumped *into* my bed, pulled the covers over my head, and had someone wake me when all the craziness was over but, I didn't. I pulled hard on my heavy comforter and my life passed before my eyes with a pain I have not experienced before.

My back seized up, I had to bend over and I couldn't breathe. I actually started moaning, screaming, AND laughing all at the same time because …well, I have no idea why I was laughing. Maybe it was to avoid swearing in front of my kids or to keep them from being scared. Anyway, my boys ran to get a neighbor and I remembered how to use my cell phone (the pain actually made me forget how to make a call!) and called my husband at work.

My neighbor, Laura, came over and she was so comforting and praying for me in Spanish. I was hunched over a couch as my children kept an eye on me and an eye out for my husband.

Rock pulled up into the driveway and then ran in and helped me to get off of the couch, down onto the floor. I said, "Call William." He called my Jin Shin Jyutsu practitioner. William did whatever energetic voo-doo he does from 15 miles away. He listened to my symptoms and said, "It's her gall bladder. It's an emotionally rooted issue and the muscles around that area are weakened. When you have a vulnerable organ, the muscles around it can get more easily strained."

He told Rock to put one hand on this part of my body and another on another part. My husband did what William said and within a few, short minutes the ripping pain in my back was gone.

I got up. I could breathe. It was almost miraculous.

Wisdoms that Saved My Bacon

I believe William was right, because I believe in the connection between emotions and sickness/dis-ease.

But I'm not the only one.

Decades ago, when you looked at an anatomical models in the medical colleges, (you know the ones, with the headless trunk of the body with the removable organs inside) you'd see that on the organs were written emotions: 'Fright' was written on the kidneys, 'Worry' on the stomach, 'Anger' on the liver, 'Offense' on the gallbladder and much more.

I was feeling offended/frustrated with a friend who was expecting a lot of me in a very busy time in my life. I felt this sense of chronic disappointment from her and a lack of understanding about all that I had going on. I was a working mom with young kids. I was on a healing journey and dealing with dizziness a lot of the time.

I was affected by the way she was treating me, but I didn't say anything. I kept swallowing this offense and, according to William, it got stuck in my gall bladder.

If you believe, as I do, that emotions can affect us physically, then maybe this resonates for you, too.

I was out of the flow with my highest self.

I was not representing *me*.

And that, over time, started affecting me.

You're Not Crazy and You're Not Alone

Through those 'holds', William helped me to restore that emotional flow, and therefore peace, to my body.

There are so many stories of how it helps with hormones, cancers, nerve issues, injuries and more. I have a link for you in the back of the book.

Honestly, I am not an expert at Jin Shin and though I have taken some classes the last few years, I'm still a newbie. BUT what I can tell you is that I regularly do what are known as 'finger holds'. In Jin Shin, they teach that each finger relates to an organ and an emotion:

- Thumb is for Worry (Stomach/Spleen)
- Pointer is for Fear (Kidney/Bladder)
- Middle Finger is for Anger (shocking I know) (Gall Bladder/ Liver)
- Ring Finger is for Sadness (Lungs and Large Intestines)
- Pinky is for 'Trying' (basically trying to do something in your own will but outside your flow) (Heart and Small Intestines)

(www.intuitiveheal.com/jsj-hand.html)

'Trying' is also described as 'pretense'. I hold this finger when I have to do an interview, or meet someone for the first time, so that I can stay true to myself and not 'try' to impress or be something I'm not.

I do it if I wake up in the middle of the night, and have something on my mind. This is my way of meditating and it brings me peace.

Gotta share ANYTHING that helps bring peace, right?

Right.

4. Grounding/Earthing

I remember learning in Psych 101 that about one hundred years ago (or as my 11 year-old says "Way Back When") in psychiatric wards there was a calming technique that was used: when a patient went into a fit, the doctors would take the patient, sit them against a tree and tie them to it.

The tree remedy calmed the patient.

Fast-forward 25 years since my college days, and the concept of 'grounding' or 'earthing' came to me as wisdom from a friend.

It is basically the idea that the earth is an electrical planet and we are bio-electrical beings who have positive and negative charges that the earth can exchange with us. With our modern culture, we tend to be more deficient in the earth's energy – staying in our shoes all day or houses all day keep us from the good energy of the earth.

Now, I know this all sounds all 'woo-woo' and that's okay. I think at this point you know that I kinda am … but in a good way so, roll with me.

When we spend time with our feet/hands/body in the grass/ sand/rocks/dirt/mud or ocean, the earth exchanges with us from its charge to ours. We get balanced from the earth. It takes the electrical charge of what is too much in us, and gives to us the balancing charge from the earth that we need.

I have been doing this for years and have to tell you, it is a calming, centering, peace-giving, and yet energizing thing to do.

According to Dr. Mercola, It also can thin your blood and reduce your blood pressure. (See: www.Mercola.com)

The earth is an amazing gift that is here to constantly give to us.

David 'Avocado' Wolfe is an inspiring health resource. When I attended his Longevity Now Conference, everyone was grounded through a device which helped people be attentive, have good posture, and stay energized throughout the long conference. So, even though I think that being out in nature is a first choice, the truth is that if you live in Alaska and have 8 months of winter where your bare feet don't get to touch green grass, there are devices that you can purchase to ground yourself while you're right inside your home. This is good stuff.

Seriously, next time you're feeling outside of yourself, try opening the door and actually going outside, put your bare feet in the earth and just breathe. I'm confident it's going to make a good and grounding difference in your life.

Wisdoms that Saved My Bacon

5. Bentonite Clay

Remember my Fettuccine Alfredo story (who can forget, right?) Well, if I had Bentonite Clay that night, I'm pretty sure I would have had a way less painful and embarrassing experience.

Bentonite Clay is a negatively charged clay that expands with water, and binds to toxins and removes them through our waste. Something I desperately needed at that dinner party.

I learned about it when my dear, sister-friend, Laurie Umbriaco (Dr. Ralph's wife) a colon hydro-therapist, told me about her food poisoning experience. She ate something awful, had a HUGE event to attend the next night, and spent the morning of the event barfing her brains out. Lovely.

She climbed into bed with a huge glass of water and her huge bottle of Sonne's Bentonite Clay and just sipped on both all day. She was able to attend the event that night. She didn't eat a whole lot, and she didn't feel fabulous, but she was significantly better because of the clay.

I bought a bottle and have been hooked ever since. Whenever the kids have a tummy ache, the flu, too much sugar at a birthday party, a dirty strawberry at the Farmer's Market or an accidental gluten exposure, I give them Bentonite. Within minutes there's relief and an ability to go poop or stop pooping -- to throw up or stop throwing up. I've found that the clay helps with whatever the body needs.

Remember the old American Express commercial, 'Don't leave home with out it'?

Yeah, well, I could do a Bentonite Clay commercial with the very same motto.

6. EMFs (Electro-Magnetic Frequencies)

The infamous summer of 2012 included having Whooping Cough.

I know. Exciting, right?

Well, we had been coughing through half of May, all of June and all of July. I must have either had an enlightening experience or lost some brain cells after sitting at home, with my children, all day, every day, with no TV and no babysitter, and no camps -- because *this* is the hair-brained, Lucy Ricardo idea I came up with: 'Let's turn off almost all of our electric breakers and live a low electricity/indoor camping experience for the month of August.'

I told the boys and my husband about the idea and mentioned two things:

1. I would blog about it throughout the month and...

2. At the end of August, we would take a special trip to the Redwoods up in Northern California.

Everyone was game, especially my husband, who goes to

work in an air-conditioned office five days a week. So, really for him - it was no big whoop.

So, we figured out how our crazy house was wired and turned every breaker off except for two. We still kept power to my husband's office computer, the refrigerator and dishwasher as well as the washer and dryer in the garage. I mean really, I wanted to have a new experience but I didn't want it to be a Little House on the Prairie, wash-my-clothes-with-a-stone-in-the-river experience. We started August 1, 2012. I quickly discovered and blogged about a couple of things:

1. How different the nighttime sounds and feels when you're not opening up a laptop, smartphone or popping in a DVD.

2. How much your family talks and holds each other when you're all centered in the living room where the candles are.

3. How early and quickly you fall asleep when there's nothing else to do.

4. How hot it really can get in August.

5. How important it is to pick up all the Lego's while it's still light out.

6. How putting a candle on the back of your toilet is a good idea in theory, until you try to sit down to go poop and nearly light yourself on fire.

You're Not Crazy and You're Not Alone

There were many more lessons than that: some profoundly deep, and some silly and light. Most were about a return to simplicity. It cultivated a deep gratitude in me – not because it reminded us of all we had with modern technology – but it reminded us of all the generosity there was to be found in nature, darkness, and silence.

It was, indeed, a rich time.

Well, we loved it so much that the boys asked if we could do it longer – and so we did. We kept going through Daylight Savings and Thanksgiving right up until December 12th when my mom arrived for a month-long visit.

Now, here's the interesting thing about December 12th: my mom arrived, my new Bloom Beautiful book arrived, and we turned a few more breakers on.

And that's when the dizziness, which I had not had in months, started back up.

We kept the breakers on for the next couple of months and I got a call from the local newspaper, and then, ABC News, asking to do an interview on our family and our low-electricity/indoor camping experiment. I said, "Sure, but we turned a couple of breakers back on for the Winter and will be turning them off again come March for Daylight Savings time."

They said: "Great!" And wanted to come by a few days after we turned them off again.

Sure enough, we did a little ritual, turned the breakers back off, and my dizziness disappeared.

I was intrigued. Dr. Barrett, my naturopath, was surprised, "Wow. I would never have pegged you to be someone who was EMF sensitive." We couldn't ignore the evidence in my life that, apparently, I was.

My friend, Joni August Brice, co-founder of Safer Technologies (www.safertech.com) has a hand-held meter that reads the EMF emissions in your home and has a product to help limit your exposure with your cell phone. Joni shared her passion and story with me:

"I've always been sensitive to energy in all its forms, and I've felt its power to affect us. I figured out that I was sensitive to electromagnetic energy when I was 19—I had no idea what an EMF was at the time, but I could just feel it. Knowing my sensitivity, I'm careful to not consume negative media and I use Jin Shin Jyutsu for healing from the affects of EMFs.

Just recently, I cut an educational video showing a dirty glass of water next to a clean one. Sure, you can drink the dirty one and you may or may not get sick. That's true. But if you choose the clean, clear water, the chances are much better that you won't get sick. Plus, you'll just feel better about the water you and your family are drinking.

Likewise, you can put the cell phone to your ear and experience all those 'waves' of radiation going into your head and some damage may or may not happen. But if you use a headset, you're creating distance from the radiation and choosing the 'cleaner' way to 'drink in' conversation and just like the clean, clear water, you feel better and you are certainly safer.

So for me, EMFs are just one more form of energy that we can be sensitive to, and that's why I'm so passionate about educating people about them, and empowering others to make informed, healthy choices in our wireless world. I've always said that I never want to be fear-driven: it's about empowering people to make the best choice for their health."

Neither Joni nor I want you to feel afraid. And I don't want you going on a witch-hunt of all the things you're possibly sensitive to. You know me by now: I'm about seeking Wisdom. I'm not about seeking the problem. As for the awareness of the EMF stuff, I just want you to feel informed and empowered.

For me, personally, I know there's a high value in keeping the lighting natural and the EMFs limited. I like life better when there's more nature and less electricity coursing through my home and my life. It allows me to breathe and feel a greater calm.

I'm truly convinced after experiencing life more au naturale, that there are great things that get brought to light while you're living in the dark.

7. Seek Wisdom

There is something very liberating and expansive about seeking Wisdom. Albert Einstein said, "You can't solve a problem with the same mind that created it."

Wisdoms that Saved My Bacon

Sometimes we just spin out with what's going on in our head or our body and we need to call on another influence to center us.

I'm going to tell you a story but, truthfully, I could tell you a hundred stories of how asking God/Spirit/The Universe for Wisdom has yielded amazing results.

I was having a strange symptom of a deeply orange tongue. Not kidding. As if someone had painted it with a Burnt Sienna Crayola crayon. It was weird.

Dizzy and an orange tongue, do not a happy life make.

My husband saw it. My kids saw it. My friends and neighbors (God bless them for looking) saw it. And I even drove across town to stick my tongue out at my doctor and say, "Thee??! Do you thee my oranthe thongue!?"

She did. I was validated.

But no one had answer. None of the doctors and nowhere on the Internet could I find a single diagnosis.

Oh god, I prayed regularly about that for a good year and a half until one day, while sitting in the tub I said, "God. I have been praying about this orange tongue for a while. Where is the Wisdom for me?"

I heard back, in Words with No Voice, 'Your Wisdom is in the unknown.' I closed my eyes to savor those words and sunk deeper into the tub, which suddenly felt like the womb of the Divine.

Wow.

At that moment, I embraced the unknown and I embraced my lack of an answer as a 'wisdom.' Even though I didn't fully understand that, it somehow made perfect sense. And once I did receive my lack of knowing – or the unknown - as a gift to me, I had this almost immediate confidence that my answer would come soon.

A few days later, a friend treated our family to a trip to Disneyland. Now, you have to know a couple of things:

1. We live twenty minutes away from Disneyland.
2. I had been dizzy with an orange tongue for a year and a half at that point.
3. Disneyland almost never feels like a 'treat' to me. But especially not when my head is in a swirl.

I'm sorry. I know I sound grumpy but I'm not. While it's a wildly creative place and Walt Disney was a genius, I just think it's overstimulating and distracting, especially to my brain, which had been dizzy for such a long time.

But the boys had gone through so much with me being so ill and our finances being so small that I said, "Yes" to the generous offer. The two little ones and the big one I married thought it would be a great idea.

Wisdoms that Saved My Bacon

So, I dubbed it our trip to "Dizzyland" and off we went.

The boys were excited to ride on Thunder Mountain with their dad and I was excited to find a bench in the shade to sit down and remember how to breathe.

I found a place next to an Asian woman. I'm not sure who put the nickel in her but the minute I sat down, she talked non-stop.

I didn't want to talk. I tried the short nods. She didn't get the hint. I tried checking my phone. Still didn't get it. Finally, something clicked in me that said, 'Listen to her. Sometimes when people talk to you and don't stop, they have a gift to give you.'

So, I turned and asked her about her native China she had been talking about. "Is it stressful there? And do people have a lot of thyroid issues because of the stress?"

I wondered about that because I know they have a diet rich in iodine, but I also wanted to inquire about the stress connection.

She seemed taken aback by my question and said, "Well, yes, it IS very stressful and we do have many thyroid issues. I know that because I am a Chinese medical doctor."

I looked in her eyes and smiled, "May I ask you a question then? Because my tongue's been orange for a year and a half and no one can figure out why."

She nodded, "Oh! That's easy!"

You're Not Crazy and You're Not Alone

Did she say "Easy?" None of my doctors for 18 months could figure ANYTHING out but she's saying it's "easy."

"Sure," she continued, "It's a blood deficiency. You need to eat green apples, meat and vegetables. Walk about 2 hours a day and take Vitamin D. It will go away."

I thanked her and thanked God and after a long day at Dizzyland, went home to start her protocol.

Within about a week of doing what she said, the orange tongue went away.

Uh. Mazing.

Wisdom is all around. Ask for it about the pain in your shoulder, the bump on your butt, the situation with your mother-in-law, the doctor you're supposed to see, the website you're supposed to find ...whatever it is.

Whether it's about Hashimoto's or some other health thing or basically anything. I believe we are invited and welcomed to seek Wisdom and that it is generously given to us. It can be in the most unexpected, delightful and even aggravating places. And, as I've learned but still don't completely understand,

Sometimes the Wisdom is even in the unknown.

Seek Wisdom.

Chapter 15

Advice to My Younger 'Me'

So, this Hashimoto's thing has been quite a journey.

If I had the ability to go back and tell my 27 year-old self some things with 20/20 hindsight, I would tell her this:

Dear Younger Me:

1. Stacey, change your diet NOW.

Eat meat, veggies, a few fruits and natural/unrefined sugar. You think you can't live without pasta and bread, you Italian-girl? You think you can't do life without all the foods you grew up on? Try living without energy and without hope and eventually you'll give up pasta and bread without blinking.

Oh, and on the subject of food: choose whole, fresh foods and pesticide-free wherever you can. And if you can't, just bless it. Don't freak out and get tweaked about every little thing, that's the kind of stress that you don't need. The power is in you, ultimately, so use your power to choose well and to bless whatever you eat.

And eat little meals every 2-3 hours. None of this waiting 7-8 hours between meals crap. Because when you don't eat for that long, it stresses out your adrenal glands and they're already hanging on by a wee little thread so, help them out and eat more regularly.

2. Rest and sleep.

Being hyper-productive is counter-productive to your healing. If you have to choose between getting one more thing done and putting yourself to bed one hour earlier -- go to bed. Even if you don't sleep (which you may not for a while), welcome the rest and let it be a meditative time for you.

3. Drink pure water.

Not all waters are created equal. Find something alkaline with good minerals. And make sure you drink enough of it – it's easy to be under-hydrated with Hashimoto's.

4. Stay away from fluoride and soy.

It sabotages your thyroid amongst other things. Fluoride is in toothpaste and water. Buy natural non-fluoride brands, even if it costs you more. It will ultimately cost you less, health-wise, in the long run. Soy is still in a lot of stuff. It pulls iodine away from your thyroid. No bueno. No eat-io or drink-io. There are big fluoride and soy bandwagons, don't get on them.

5. Heal your heart.

There's stuff from the past that you need to work out that's tormenting you, and has set negative beliefs in place. This stuff needs to be addressed. You need your mind, body and spirit to work for you, and not against you when you're healing. Get help with this and keep on your heart-healing journey. You're worth the work.

6. Release toxic people.

You're in a sensitive time and you know it. You don't need those negative, critical people in your life to dump their 'everything is impossible' mindset on you. And you don't need to hang out with folks who are hyper-critical of you, either. Stick with folks who know how to see the sunny side of things and the best side of you.

Spend your time with people who love you and aren't focused on judging you. Letting toxic folks go is part of your healing and an expression of your self-love.

7. Do gentle exercise.

Gone are your days of hours of aerobics and heavy weight lifting … at least for a while. Gentle walks, lighter weights, and yoga do something different to your mitochondria and are a non-stressful way to move your body. You need as much of that 'non-stressful' stuff as you can while you're healing.

8. Listen to your body and your intuition.

You were given an inner compass and sense of direction. You may feel like you lost it, but it's just been suppressed with all you've gone through in life.

Practice listening again.

What everyone else does, eats and drinks may not be right for you, so keep your inner inquiry going and listen to how you feel. If you're tired after you eat, that food's not right for you. If you're depressed after you eat, that food doesn't work. If you're moody after you eat, that food isn't your friend.

Your body is your ally, not your enemy -- being disconnected from it and overworking it didn't serve you so, start listening to it again and re-establishing your connection to yourself.

9. Liver, Adrenals, Thyroid, and Gut are all connected.

Learn about the connection between your liver, your adrenals, your thyroid and your gut. If you take care of your liver, your thyroid is happier. If you take care of your adrenals, your thyroid is much happier. If you take care of your gut, your thyroid is so happy it practically wants to throw a parade. The Liver, Adrenals, and Gut are the essential and supporting cast for the Thyroid. Without them, the show does not go on.

10. The doctors aren't the final word.

There are great doctors out there. And then, there are doctors who are not right for you. I'm talking about the latter right now: they may look at your labs or look at you and tell you things like, "Surgery is the only way!" Or "You'll never have kids!" or "This medicine is the industry standard for your disease." And they may be wrong.

Step back and take an inventory. If the person isn't life-giving and won't work with you in a peer-like, mutually respectful way, step back. You will be tempted to blame them once you learn more but, look at them like they are just the Orange Cones in life telling you, in their own way, "Go around me -- I don't have the answer."

If you can keep from people-pleasing *for* them and holding a grudge *against* them, you will benefit from the goodness that's *within* them. And you'll be able to hear when something doesn't ring true for you. Keep looking, there's an answer just for you, even if it's not with that particular doctor.

11. **Keep an open mind, do research, and then listen to your inner wisdom.**

As you step toward the natural healing world, people will have many different ideas about what's best for you. What may work for someone else doesn't necessarily mean it will work for you.

You will be tempted to think that the next remedy or treatment for a thousand dollars or ten thousand dollars is your only hope. But take a second to breathe. Do a little research, and listen to that inner voice.

I'm not saying to be guarded and judgmental, or to think everyone's out to screw you (which is the other end where the pendulum swings after you think people are your Obi-Wan). I'm just saying you don't have to jump on every bandwagon. Be wise.

12. Write in your journal.

There is so much that you're going to process through. Write it down.

Do those morning pages that Julia Cameron talks about in The Artist's Way: stream of consciousness for three hand-written pages when you wake up. It will clear the deck of your brain and leave space for creative solutions in your health and your life. You will see certain patterns you didn't realize or issues that really matter to you. It will be a place where release happens and dreams manifest.

Also, keep a symptoms journal. Write the date and what kind of food you're eating, sleep you're getting and poop you're pooping. Brain fog isn't the best for remembering important details so, give yourself the gift of keeping a journal.

13. Go to nature.

Nature is your friend. Put your feet in the earth or the sand or the ocean. Take that time to ground yourself. Technology is great as a tool to serve you and your research. But don't make it your only pastime or your default to distract you from what's really going on in life. Because sitting in front of a computer all day isn't what feeds your soul.

Nature is progressively and consistently healing itself. So go out, be in nature, and align with it. It will settle you, give you perspective and help you to breathe (you hold your breath a lot you know.)

Breathe.

14. Save your Adrenal Glands.

If stress feels peaceful and peace feels stressful, that's a pretty good sign that you're living off of your Adrenal Glands.

Those little guys have been through a lot. All the stress from growing up, the stress of going through the marriage stuff and the having kids stuff and the God stuff. Oh yeah, and the Hashimoto's stuff.

How could we forget that...

Your adrenal glands are supposed to be used for emergencies in life, not a life full of emergencies. Stress, unaddressed and unconquered makes your body feel like there's a 5-alarm fire – all. the. time.

Because of that, choose what you watch and read with care.

The last thing you need to do in your spare time, to help you 'unwind,' is viewing the news, reading drama-heavy books, and watching action-packed intense movies.

Watching those TV shows that take place in a hospital or a courtroom or a deserted island is counter-productive to your health. All those post-apocalyptic adventures? Yeah, none of them make your adrenal glands happy, Stacey.

You're a sensitive soul who needs more peace and rest and a lot less overstimulation. Don't spend your real-life energy for pretend storylines or situations you can't do anything about. Your subconscious mind doesn't know the difference and you take everything in so deeply.

Save your adrenal glands for the big things, in real life. Then, when you need them, they'll be there for you.

15. Have sex anyway.

Okay, so here's the deal: you know how much you love sex? You may go through a time where you want to put a lock over your coochie and throw away the key. Stress, kids, and lack of sleep, as well as an underactive thyroid, may threaten to take the va-va-voom out of your bedroom.

It's okay. I'm telling you now: have sex anyway.

You'll still have a connecting, good time if you let yourself. It's good for your marriage. It's good for your soul. It's the closest thing to exercise you're going to be doing for a while and your guy loves it.

He's not looking at your cellulite. Hell, he can't even find the ketchup when it's the only thing in the fridge. No, really. Seriously, I read an article about how men don't even really see cellulite the way we do. I wish I had known that when I was your age.

So, you've gained some weight. So, you're not feeling 'into' it. So, you're tired.

You're going to feel that way anyway until you sort out some of the health stuff, you might as well have some skin-on-skin time. It's good for your heart, it's going to give you some endorphins (which you probably desperately need), and heck, you may even lose some weight and get a nap out of the whole deal afterward.

This whole 'have sex anyway' can really be a good thing if you let it.

Let it.

16. Keep your identity.

You are not this dis-ease, so don't label yourself and define yourself by it.

Understand it, be an advocate of your self within it, but don't mentally become a victim to it. And have wisdom around others who have an autoimmune thing, so that it doesn't become a club of victims like crabs in a bucket: where one's always pulling down the one who's climbing higher. Be sure it's a community of support and not a bucket full of crabs.

Keep your highest goal: healing, and a rich, meaningful life. And keep your highest vibration: living in love, health, wisdom, and peace and encouraging others to do the same.

You already believe that anything is possible with Love so, stay focused on that. Healing is possible. No matter what anyone says.

You've always been a pioneer, seeing things and knowing

things before your time. You don't need agreement. Keep listening to the Wisdom within you and walk in that, no matter who agrees or applauds or argues.

17. Love yourself.

When you lose sight on the days when it's hard, ask yourself one question: 'what would I do right now if I truly loved myself?' The answer will come. And it won't be about performing for your friends, or trying to make your scoffing family understand that you're not really lazy. And it won't be about moving forward your career that you feel behind on.

Remember this: you are only a few days or a few weeks away from feeling differently. One food eliminated can make you feel better in a matter of days. One supplement, or correctly implemented remedy can make you feel better in a few weeks. Hang in there.

Be kind to you.

Don't wait for life, or you, to be perfect before you extend that kindness to yourself.

Love yourself through these bumpy times.

18. Keep your sense of humor.

There's nothing like a relentless struggle with your health to wear down your funny bone. Keep your sense of humor.

And I'm not talking about the self-deprecating kind that is always putting you and the size of your butt down. I'm talking about that stuff that makes you laugh so hard, you just about pee in your pants. The things that make your stomach hurt and make you sound like Deputy Dog because you can't catch your breath.

I put on hilarious comedian, John Pinette's "I'm Starvin'" DVD or Wayne Brady's talented antics on "Whose Line is it Anyway?" – or I read something from favorite funny writer, Jenny Lawson at her website: www.bloggess.com.

That kind of stuff? It's pure gold to you.

Laughter is healing. So, take your 'medicine.'

19. Say "No" to the good stuff.

Girl, you're funny and fun to be with. Your friends love being with you and there are so many people who want to hang out with you and your wisdom.

Don't let those times be the shiny objects that you run after. Just because someone wants to be with you doesn't mean that's where it's best for you to spend your energy.

Start listening to what your body can handle and prioritize your rest over your popularity.

I have a theory that our thyroid has waved the little white flag, partially because you never learned how to say, "No," and honor yourself. Don't make your thyroid, or your exhaustion, or your health speak for you. Be your own advocate of your time and health and use your real voice. People will survive. You'll still have friends. They will get over their disappointment, and you will get over your own disappointment in their disappointment. (That's called 'guilt', by the way, and it's not your friend.)

Be a "Yes!" to you by saying, "No!" to what doesn't serve your ultimate good.

You are worth the "Yes!"

20. Be in Gratitude.

It will be tempting to be resentful and compare yourself at this age and this energy level to where others are. It will also be tempting to compare yourself to the dreams you had for your life. You'll be tempted to ask, 'Where did my 20's and 30's go?' This will not serve you or your healing to compare yourself to anyone or where you thought you'd be by now.

This is where you are. It's not *who* you are, but it's *where* you are. If you will get yourself to a place -- past the anger and the honest yet, understandable frustration – to where you can choose gratitude, this journey will completely shift for you.

21. Keep seeking Wisdom.

It's there for you. Ask the Divine and keep your eyes open. This health journey that looked daunting at first, will become one of your most profound adventures you will take in your life. It will be full of stories that will encourage you and others deeply, and connect you to the most amazing people. Every-

Advice to My Younger 'Me'

one has a path; this is yours.

You're not alone.

Wisdom and Love are with you always.

Love,

The Older, Wiser and a tad-Saggier, but much-Happier,

Stacey

Chapter 16

How Do You Eat An Elephant (Sized Buffet)?

So, you've read the whole book, been completely touched, had many aha moments, and looking at yourself in the mirror moments and now, you're like, 'Holy Crap, where do I even begin?'

First of all, let me tell you: congratulations! You've already begun.

You've already made commitments in your heart and mind and digested a lot of stuff. It may take some time for more of it to sink in. You might be thinking, 'Wait! I'm 300 lbs and I want to be 150!' or 'Oh no, I'm not even sure I can live without gluten let alone try the whole AIP!' (Autoimmune Paleo Protocol)

Trust me I get it.

When I start feeling overwhelmed, like there's too much to do and too far to go in this whole thing, I often get a picture of a buffet. You know like one of the grand, million-miles-of-food things they have in Las Vegas or fancy resorts – *that* kind of buffet.

And I think to myself, 'I'm overwhelmed because I'm trying to eat this whole buffet like it's a one-course meal.'

You're Not Crazy and You're Not Alone

And that's just not possible to do. So don't even try.

Remember Marla Cilley from The FLYLady who did ONE new thing a MONTH? And in nine months she had a system down that transformed her life and the lives of millions of women.

With my thyroid journey for the last 17 years, I can share this bit of wisdom with you: it's like that question: "How do you eat an elephant?"

The answer is: one bite at a time.

How do you take on your life and this Hashimoto's thing? One choice at a time.

It's tempting to look at people who are feeling stronger, are thriving at gluten-free, are exercising again or, holy crap, are actually *losing* weight! And you're still just trying to get out of bed in the morning, feeling that mix of hoping you don't die, but wishing you were dead.

There are so many phases to this thing that it can feel like an elephant in just the massive size alone: dealing with exhaustion, the letting go of overworking, first physically and then, mentally - and then, relationally.

Then, it goes on but not necessarily in this order:

- Letting go of toxic people and thoughts.
- Letting go of the guilt of how you can't perform the way you used to and who that's affecting (like kids, partner, parents, friends, co-workers, etc...)

How to Eat an Elephant-Sized Buffet

- Then, letting go of toxic foods and patterns.

And that's just the Letting Go section. We haven't even talked about the Adding Things section.

- Adding things like medicine or supplements or both.
- Adding gentle exercise.
- Adding healing liquids.
- Adding healing remedies.

And allowing yourself to dream again when you weren't even sure you were going to make it through the day, let alone have a future to dream into.

Overwhelmed yet?

Or what about those times when you're making great strides, and then you get brave (or ridiculous) enough and try an old food too soon. Or you work too much and start feeling crappy again. You're facing how you're going to deal with that repair mode without losing hope...

again.

It's so much.

I want you to know something: you can do this.

All that stuff is overwhelming if you're trying to deal with it like it's a one-course meal. That's why I talk about seeking Wisdom. I believe that Wisdom will lead you to the priority of which thing to put on your plate for this season.

You're Not Crazy and You're Not Alone

We're all here to share where we are as we sit at the table togeth-er. Some are on their first trip up to the buffet and feeling that mix of overwhelmed, scared, and excited. Some are in the middle of the journey on the pineapple and cottage cheese round (seri-ously, who does that, I mean, really...) and getting their mojo back. And some are already onto the dessert part of the whole thing really feeling like they can live a great life while traveling with the diagnosis of Hashimoto's.

There's a great big community to share the table, with amazing people right beside you, here to encourage you.

There's more help than there ever was.

Thank you, to all the amazing people, Facebook groups, web-sites, doctors, health professionals, family, and friends who are there to support and strengthen folks with Hashimoto's and oth-er autoimmune dis-eases. You are Amazing Love and a comfort to those of us who are up at night with insomnia (again) hunting and pecking on the computer in the dark, looking for someone to tell us that we're loved and we're going to be okay.

Looking for someone to remind us, that just because we feel this badly, doesn't mean that it's the end. And, just because it seems like we'll never feel good again, doesn't mean that we won't.

When we're in that place where it feels like it's all going to pot, you've been there to remind us:

We're not crazy
And we're not alone.

How to Eat an Elephant-Sized Buffet

Let me be another voice of Love telling you:

You're not.
And you're not.

Okay, well, you might be a *little* bit crazy.

But not in that bad-crazy way. I mean in that crazy-good way that the world needs you to be and wouldn't be the same without you. The unique thing you bring, and the way you think, and the way you love.

I'm so glad you're here.
You are so important to this conversation
And your life makes a difference in this life.

Don't lose hope. You chose this book for a reason. You know your purpose here is great.

You just needed a little reminder, like we all do from time to time:

You're what the world's been waiting for.

I would love to hear your stories about how
You're Not Crazy and You're Not Alone
has impacted *your* life.

Please contact me:

Email: contact@staceyrobbins.com
Facebook: www.facebook.com/staceyrobbins

I'm excited to hear from you!

- Stacey

Gratitudes

For the friends who have my back and my heart, no matter what project I'm working on: You make this whole 'breathing in and out' thing called 'Life' one of the best places to be: Angela Ippolito, Ken Tamplin, Laurie Umbriaco, Carissa Boles, Irene Dunlap, Hope Hokama, Joni Brice, Susannah Parrish, and Tracy Panzarella.

For the devoted and unbelievable support, with an 18-hour time change thrown in, just for giggles: Danielle Pearsall, I'm beyond grateful for how you stood for this project and for me as well as for your research and assistance on the Referrals page. You rock. No, really. You do.

For the Facebook group, Hashimotos411: This community, founded by Alice Berry McDonnell and maintained by such beautiful, passionate and amazing women was a place where I was able to share these ideas which were so warmly received. Many of the women would ask me, "Stacey, when are you writing a book? We need this!" The answer is now. And it's for you. Thank you!

For David Trotter: Book layout and design master-guru-person, massively supportive friend with a generous heart, I'm so grateful for our friendship – Thank you!

For Lance and Lyndia Leonard and Linda Masterson: We've known each other a short time and yet, forever. I feel your good energy and support in palpable ways. Your love makes me strong and I'm so very grateful.

New friends and mentors: April Morris and Darlene Willman: This book was birthed after my commitment merged with yours. This flowed and magic happened. Love that. So glad our lives have intersected for the good work we're here to do. Thank you!

For the prayers and natural healing wisdom of my Mom: She was always bent more toward the holistic way of doing things. I love that it not only serves me, but will serve my children and their children and on and on...so grateful and I love you. Thank you, Mom!

For my husband, Rock: Who believes in me when life is unbelievable and blesses me when I'm beyond cranky. (Which, as you and I know, honey, *rarely* happens. Ahem...) Your love and deep kindness make a difference in my life. There's no one I'd rather be bored with or travel the globe with (or anything between with) than you. Thank you for believing in me. I love you and believe in you. (I know, I know, I just wrote 'believe' like a million times. So, sue me.)

To my boys, Caleb and Seth: You are divine expressions of Love. You are. And you're funny. Holy crow, you make me laugh 'til I about pee in my pants, and you help me see life in the most profoundly honest ways. Your love heals me and you know what? I'm going to spread that all around so that others are healed, too. Look at what you've done just by being you. You're freakin' amazing. And like I always say, "I may not be perfect, but I'm perfect for you." I'm so deeply, truly, unbelievably grateful to be your Mom.

Recommendations and Referrals

Health Practitioners and Healers

Dr. Ralph Umbriaco, DC
dr.ralph@mac.com
(949) 645-8320

Dr. Brett Jacques, ND
www.newportlongevitycenter.com
yolie@newportlongevitycenter.com
(949) 630-0304

Dr. Koren Barrett, ND
www.newportintegrativehealth.com
drbarrett@npihealth.com
(949) 743-5770

Dr. Izabella Wentz, PharmD., FASCP
www.thyroidlifestyle.com

Dr. Marc Ryan, LAC
www.hashimotoshealing.com
(310) 831-2202

Dr. Peter Osbourne, DC
www.towncenterwellness.com
(281) 240-2229

Dr. David Brownstein, MD
www.drbrownstein.com
(248) 851-1600

Dr. Alan Christianson, ND
www.integrativehealthcare.com
(480) 657-0003

Dr. Sara Gottfried, MD
www.saragottfriedmd.com

Dr. Mark Starr, MD
www.21centurymed.com
(480) 607-6503

Dr. Sherri Tenpenny, DO, AOBNMM, ABIHM
www.tenpennyimc.com
info@tenpennyimc.com
(440) 239-3438

Dr. Mick Hall, ND
www.35forlife.com
(714) 485-2299

Dr. Prudence Broadwell, LAC
(714) 965-9266

Recommendations and Referrals

Paige Adams, FNP, B-C
www.proactivemed.org
info@proactivemed.org
(615) 331-1973

Dr. Silvana Balsimelli, DC
(714) 556-3030

David "Avocado" Wolfe
www.davidwolfe.com

Helena Guerrera
www.biomagnetismusa.com
(707) 642-7700

Moshe Fuhrman
www.csconversations.com
(714) 323-5303

Blythe Fair
blythefairjsj@gmail.com
(949) 718-3530

Dr. Michael L. Johnson
www.youcanbeatthyroiddisorders.com
mljohnson@askdrjohnson.com
(920) 739-6971

Books

Hashimoto's Thyroiditis: Lifestyle Interventions for Finding and Treating the Root Cause
Dr. Izabella Wentz

Living Well With Hypothyroidism - What Your Doctor Doesn't Tell You... That You Need To Know
Mary Shomon

You Can Heal Your Life
Louise Hay

Adrenal Fatigue, the 21st Century Stress Syndrome
Dr. James Wilson

Why Do I Still Have Thyroid Symptoms?
Datis Kharrazian

The Complete Idiot's Guide to Thyroid Disease
Alan Christianson

The Hormone Cure
Sarah Gottfried

The 7 Principals of Fat Burning
Dr. Eric Berg

Recommendations and Referrals

Women's Bodies, Women's Wisdom
Dr. Christiane Northrup

Hypothyroidism Type 2: The Epidemic
Mark Starr

All Your Thyroid Problems Solved
Dr. Sandra Cabot

How I Reversed My Hashimoto's Thyroiditis Hypothyroidism
Robert Dirgo

A Course In Miracles
acim.org

Women, Food & God
Geneen Roth

A More Excellent Way: Be in Health
Henry W. Wright

Beautiful Inside and Out: Conquering Thyroid Disease with a Healthy, Happy, "Thyroid Sexy" Life
Gena Lee Nolin

Apple Cider Vinegar: Miracle Health System
Patricia and Paul Bragg

Online Resources

BioLumina Spirulina
newphoenixrising.com/LoveYourHealth

Hashimoto's 411
facebook.com/groups/hashimotos411/members

Elimination/Provocation Diet: Hashimoto's 411
facebook.com/groups/EPDiet411/members

Mary Shomon
stopthethyroidmadness.com

Dr. Christiane Northrup M.D & Author
facebook.com/DrChristianeNorthrup

Dr. Izabella Wentz
www.facebook.com/ThyroidLifestyle

Truth Calkins
facebook.com/ThyroidHealth

Thyroid Sexy / Gena Lee Nolin
facebook.com/thyroidsexy

The Complete Idiot's Guide to Thyroid Disease
Dr. Alan Christianson
facebook.com/ThyroidDisease

Mary Shomon
facebook.com/thyroidsupport

Hashimoto's Australia
facebook.com/groups/highlandvalley/members

Recommendations and Referrals

**FTPO - For Thyroid Patients Only
(T3 and/or CT3M Discussion Group)**
facebook.com/groups/FTPOThyroid

FTPO – UK/Europe (For Thyroid Patients Only)
facebook.com/groups/FTPOUKandEurope

Dana Trentini – Hypothyroid Mom
hypothyroidmom.com

Alanna Kaivalya
mindbodygreen.com/0-6872/How-I-Cured-an-Incurable-Disease

Thyroid Change
facebook.com/groups/thyroidchange

Underactive Thyroid Awareness
facebook.com/groups/306937466859

Jin Shin Jyutsu
facebook.com/groups/jsjphysiophilosophy
flowsforlife.com

International Paleo Movement Group
facebook.com/groups/116409718456748

Thyroid Support Group
facebook.com/groups/thyroidsupport/members

Cynthia Occelli
beautifullifeschool.com

Dan Koifman
facebook.com/groups/circadianbiohackers

You're Not Crazy and You're Not Alone

The Thyroid Support Group
groups.yahoo.com/neo/groups/The_Thyroid_Support_Group/info

The Water Brewery
thewaterbrewery.com

Dr. Masaru Emoto
masaru-emoto.net/english

Sara Gottfried
saragottfriedmd.com/blog

ThyroPhoenix
thyrophoenix.com

Joni Brice
safertech.com/team/joni-august-brice

Wellnessmama
wellnessmama.com

Green Smoothie Girl
greensmoothiegirl.com

Blenditandmendit
blenditandmendit.com

Wellness Warrior
wellnesswarrior.com

Lydia Joy Shatney
divinehealthfromtheinsideout.com

Sarah Wilson
sarahwilson.com.au/category/autoimmune

Recommendations and Referrals

Chris Kresser
chriskresser.com

Crazy Thyroid Lady
crazythyroidlady.blogspot.com.au

Stacey Thureen
staceythureen.com
thyroid.answers.com

How Not To Be A Dick To A Sick Friend
xojane.com/issues/how-not-to-be-a-dick-to-your-sick-friend

EarthClinic Home Remedies Body's pH
the basics on alkalinity and acidity
earthclinic.com/CURES/pH.html

For an updated listing of resources, see
www.staceyrobbins.com

To enjoy more of Stacey's inspiring way of looking at life:

www.bloombeautiful.com

You can order her **Bloom Beautiful** book
for yourself and the women you love.

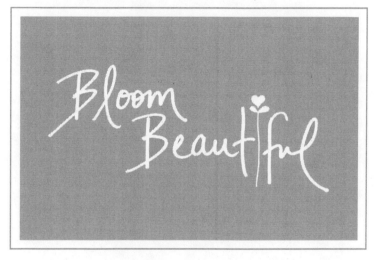

And, be sure to download her
Bloom Beautiful iPhone / iPad app
in the App Store.

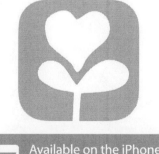

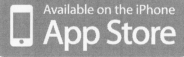

Made in the USA
San Bernardino, CA
16 February 2014